THE
POWER
FOODS
DIET

THE POWER FOODS DIET

The Breakthrough Plan That
Traps, Tames, and Burns Calories
for Easy and Permanent Weight Loss

NEAL D. BARNARD, MD, FACC

With Menus and Recipes by
DUSTIN HARDER *and* **LINDSAY S. NIXON**

balance

NEW YORK   BOSTON

Balance
Hachette Book Group
1290 Avenue of the Americas
New York, NY 10104
GCP-Balance.com
Twitter.com/GCPBalance
Instagram.com/GCPBalance

First Edition: March 2024

Balance is an imprint of Grand Central Publishing. The Balance name and logo are trademarks of Hachette Book Group, Inc.

The publisher is not responsible for websites (or their content) that are not owned by the publisher.

The Hachette Speakers Bureau provides a wide range of authors for speaking events. To find out more, go to hachettespeakersbureau.com or email HachetteSpeakers@hbgusa.com.

Balance books may be purchased in bulk for business, educational, or promotional use. For information, please contact your local bookseller or the Hachette Book Group Special Markets Department at special.markets@hbgusa.com.

Library of Congress Cataloging-in-Publication Data has been applied for.

ISBNs: 978-1-5387-6495-4 (Hardcover); 978-1-5387-6497-8 (ebook)

Printed in the United States of America

LSC-C

Printing 1, 2024

A Note to the Reader

This book will introduce you to powerful new concepts about putting the power of food to work. It's easy, and the payoff is huge, as you will soon see! Even so, let me mention two important points:

- **If you have a health condition or use medications, see your health care provider.** Often, when people improve their diets, they need less medication for diabetes, high blood pressure, or other conditions. Sometimes, they can discontinue their drugs altogether. But do not change your medications on your own. Work with your health care provider to reduce or discontinue your medicines if and when the time is right.
- **Get complete nutrition.** Include a variety of vegetables, fruits, whole grains, and legumes in your routine, and I would suggest a special focus on leafy green vegetables. Be sure to have a reliable source of vitamin B_{12} daily, such as a simple B_{12} supplement or fortified cereals or fortified soy milk. Vitamin B_{12} is essential for healthy nerves and healthy blood. You will find more details in chapter 5.

Acknowledgments

Thank you to the thousands of participants in our research studies and to Hana Kahleova, MD, PhD, and the research team of the Physicians Committee for Responsible Medicine, who have helped establish the power of healthful foods for weight loss and for many other health issues. Thank you to Gerald Shulman, MD, PhD, and Kitt Petersen, MD, at Yale University, for providing magnetic resonance spectroscopy and inspiration as we explore the power of foods.

Thanks to Dustin Harder and Lindsay S. Nixon for their culinary genius and for translating nutrition science into delicious, easy, and quick recipes that maximize weight loss and overall health. Thank you to Stefanie and the Ignoffo family, Jasmine, Shauné, Janelle, Dr. Steven Lome, and Chuck Carroll for sharing your inspiring experiences. Thank you to Carla Slajchert, L. J. Steinig, Christine Loeffler, Patty Herflicker, Sunshine Harder, Jill Eckart, Abby Power, Betsy Wason, Dania DePas, Stephanie McBurnett, Kim Kilbride, Abigail Nickerson, Tatiana Znayenko-Miller, Olly Swyers, Elizabeth Baker, Phoebe Woodruff, Emily Anderson, Noah Praamsma, and Roxie Becker for testing the recipes carefully. Thanks also to Cael Croft for the excellent diagrams. I am very grateful to all of you! Thank you to my literary agent, Brian DeFiore, for endless wisdom, guidance, and expertise, and to my editors, Nana K. Twumasi and Natalie Bautista, as well as the Hachette team for their collaboration in creating this book.

Contents

Recipe Table of Contents

Desserts

Staples, Condiments, and Dressings

Introduction

You are about to learn the easiest and most effective way to lose weight permanently. It's easy, because foods will do the work for you. You will not go hungry. You will not need to count calories or fear carbohydrates. You will not even need to exercise unless, of course, you want to.

Three scientific breakthroughs made this possible:

1. Appetite-Taming Foods. The first breakthrough occurred in 2005. Our research team at the Physicians Committee for Responsible Medicine in Washington, DC, found that certain foods are remarkably effective at taming the appetite. The research study included sixty-four women who wanted to lose weight. We found that certain foods caused them to feel so full and satisfied that, without realizing it, they were eating hundreds fewer calories per day than before and losing weight easily. They lost about a pound per week, week after week, without intentionally reducing portions or exercising.[1] The research team then followed the participants for two additional years, finding that, as long as they put the right foods to work, the lost weight never came back. That is because the appetite-taming effect works indefinitely. In later studies, we have confirmed this finding, as have other research teams. By focusing on certain healthy foods, participants who normally eat 2,000 calories or more per day felt full and satisfied eating far fewer calories.

Only later did we realize that certain foods have the same appetite-reducing action as the prescription drugs Ozempic and Wegovy, which have recently become popularized for weight loss. These foods trigger the release of a natural compound called GLP-1, which signals the brain to stop eating, but without the risks or expense of prescription drugs. Surprised? You will learn all about that here.

2. Calorie-Trapping Foods. The second breakthrough came in 2017. Tufts University researchers found that certain foods trap calories in the digestive tract and escort them out with the waste.[2] These *calorie-trapping* foods allow you to eat normal amounts and then literally flush calories away.

This is an astounding idea. If you were to eat, say, 500 calories at a meal, you would think that you would absorb 500 calories. And you will, if you eat like most people do. However, by selecting certain foods detailed in this book, some of those calories are trapped, so they cannot be absorbed.

3. Calorie-Burning Foods. The third breakthrough came in 2020, when our research team proved that certain foods are *metabolism boosters*. They increase your calorie-burning speed for hours after every meal.[3] That means a portion of their calories are simply burned and cannot be stored as fat. As you will see, these simple, healthful foods actually change what is happening inside your cells, boosting your calorie-burning ability.

Power Foods

Certain foods give you all three effects *at the same time*: These power foods tame your appetite, trap and flush calories away, and boost your metabolism simultaneously. As a result, this approach is extremely effective for weight loss—more so than if you were to lace up your sneakers and run every day of your life, or if you were to measure and limit every morsel you consumed.

These three breakthroughs were then followed by more discoveries.

It turns out that natural compounds in everyday foods, like blueberries, cinnamon, mangoes, apples, and many others, boost weight loss even more. We now know how to put them to work.

Sometimes the power of these foods is referred to as a "negative calorie effect." That does not mean the foods have no calories—or fewer than none; it means, of however many calories a food may hold, a sizable number are subtracted by the food's ability to flush calories away before they can be absorbed or to release them as body heat, so they cannot be stored as fat. That means certain foods make weight loss easy. The more these foods are in your routine, the more you lose.

Our research participants have found other benefits, too. They have more energy, their skin looks healthier, their cholesterol levels improve, their overall health rebounds, and they sleep better.

Delicious and Powerful

Imagine starting your day with waffles topped with blueberry syrup, and finishing it with a delicious penne arrabbiata, never worrying about calories or carbohydrates, and losing weight whether you exercise or not. If you are pressed for time or just prefer not to cook, you will see how easy it is to include power foods in your routine.

This book presents research findings from many universities and research centers, including our own studies at the Physicians Committee in Washington, DC. Much of what you read here will be totally new to you, but, if you follow the guidance in this book, you will never diet again, you will never count calories, and you will never go to bed hungry.

New, Different, and Empowering

Before going further, let me make one thing clear: Weight gain is not the result of a moral failing or weak willpower. It is not your fault. The fact is, without you knowing it, certain less than healthy foods have altered your body's metabolic balance in an unhelpful way. Your appetite has expanded, and your metabolism has probably slowed down over time. This is a common experience. But no matter how long you have been struggling with weight issues, you can now use healthful foods to reset your balance.

Most people have no idea about the real power that foods have—or which foods help and which ones hurt. As they gain weight, they resort to punishing diets—diets with near-starvation portions, diets that ban "carbs" and make you feel guilty for wanting a piece of bread or fruit, diets that restrict you to one meal a day, and diet programs that charge for meals week after week after week. You will be free of all that.

In this book, you will explore a broad range of delicious foods that you can put to work to lose weight and improve your overall health. You will have a treasury of menus and recipes developed by two premier culinary experts, Dustin Harder and Lindsay S. Nixon. Dustin is a chef and author who leads culinary programs for the Physicians Committee. Lindsay is a bestselling author whose recipes have been featured in the *New York Times, Shape, Fitness,* and *Women's Health,* and on *WebMD.* Both have a knack for building powerful weight-loss ingredients into healthful, delicious recipes. They will share their secrets with you.

You will learn easy and quick food preparation techniques you can use at home, and you will instantly know which foods are the best choices at the grocery store or at restaurants. If you are allergic to cooking and rely on convenience foods, I will show you your best choices.

Although this book is founded on carefully done scientific research, you will find the explanations simple and the program easy to follow. It will also help you cut through the noise. There is a lot of hype about various foods these days: Often a headline about the "health benefits" of a certain food or nutritional supplement turns out to be based on very thin science—an experiment using mice or a single observational study with no other evidence. In some cases, experiments are funded by supplement manufacturers who are trying to make marketing claims. This book carefully sifts through the evidence.

Along the way, you will not only have a chance to try new tastes and have fun with delicious foods, you will also be able to reach a level of health that you had perhaps thought was unattainable. Our research team has been studying the best food choices, not just for weight loss, but also for tackling diabetes, cholesterol, high blood pressure, menstrual symptoms, menopausal hot flashes, and joint pain, and we have identified the best choices for athletic performance, sexual vitality, and long-term cognitive health.

This approach is empowering, exciting, and life-changing. Let's jump in.

PART 1

HOW FOODS CAUSE WEIGHT LOSS

CHAPTER 1

The Breakthroughs and What They Mean for You

In this chapter, we'll explore how foods trim away weight naturally. Once you know the basic principles, you can put them to work at home, when you shop for food, and when you dine out. In the following chapters, we will look at which foods are your best choices, as well as foods that can slow down your progress and are best avoided.

Our team has been conducting research studies since the 1990s. Funded by the National Institutes of Health, we revolutionized the approach to diabetes, laying the groundwork for viewing type 2 diabetes as a potentially reversible condition for many patients. We have done the same for cholesterol problems, menopausal symptoms, and other everyday conditions. Each of these breakthroughs has led to a complete rethinking about how foods affect our bodies. This book is about breakthroughs for weight loss that provide the safest and most effective method yet available.

To give you a feel for how these breakthroughs came about, I would like to tell part of this story through the experiences of our research participants. They come into our research center for tests of various kinds, and we get together weekly so they can learn how to put foods to work and so we can track their progress. In relating these experiences, I will invite you to learn along with them.

Let me first introduce you to a research volunteer named Liz. Liz was, and still is, an attorney for the US government. She was in her early thirties when the study began, and her work kept her on the run. She had always tried to eat a more or less healthful diet but had not been able to reach her goal weight. She had tried various diets, but their effects were mostly short-term and more modest than she was looking for. She joined our research study because she liked the idea of a science-based approach and felt that it would give her some structure and support.

The research team told her about foods that *cause* weight loss. They were familiar foods, although not necessarily foods she ate frequently. She put them to work, favoring certain ones and avoiding others. The very first week, she saw the results on her scale, and weight loss continued week after week. Using a special DEXA (dual-energy X-ray absorbtiometry) scanner, our team tracked exactly how much fat she had lost from her abdomen, hips, and everywhere else.

Along the way, her health improved enormously. Her chronic indigestion—acid stomach—went away. Her cholesterol improved. Her mood was better, and she had more energy. Her friends remarked about how good she looked.

At the moment, Liz is on a train headed from Washington, DC, to New Haven, Connecticut. She has just about finished the study and is bursting with excitement. She has finally conquered her problem with some surprisingly easy tricks. Now she was headed to Yale University to help the research team answer one last question: How is it that foods could work this magic—what had changed inside her body?

Arriving in New Haven, Liz made her way to a buzzing medical center, where special scanning equipment would allow the researchers to look *inside her cells*. That is where the answer would be found, or so they hoped.

At the magnetic resonance spectroscopy suite, a technician asked Liz to put on a gown and lie on a table next to what looked like an enormous plastic doughnut. The technician made sure she was comfortable, then flipped a switch. Gradually, the table slid into the doughnut hole, carrying her with it. As she lay inside the magnetic resonance scanner, the research team examined her muscle cells, liver cells, and parts of her cellular makeup that would influence how fast she burned calories. And, yes, it turned out that simple food choices had changed her fundamental body chemistry.

Shortly, you'll learn about the changes they found in Liz's cells, why weight loss had suddenly become easy for her, and what it means for *your* cells, *your* body, *your* weight, and *your* health. But first let's go back to the beginning so you can understand how we got here.

Discovering the Appetite-Taming Effect

Long before the research study that Liz had volunteered for, our team published the surprising results of another study in the *American Journal of Medicine*.[1] The research volunteers were women with weight problems, some severe. They had tried a great many diets without success. Low-calorie, low-carbohydrate, meal-replacement bars, cabbage soup—you name it, they had tried it.

Our approach was different. Rather than focusing on *how much* they ate, we helped the women change *what* they ate, with a special emphasis on foods that satisfy the appetite with fewer calories. Indeed, we found that the participants pushed away from the table having taken in a couple of hundred calories less than usual. Without any intentional limitations on calories or portions, they lost about a pound a week. We then tracked the participants for two additional years, finding that the slimming effect kept going indefinitely.

We did a similar study with the GEICO insurance company, which invited company employees who wanted to lose weight or improve their health to learn about healthier foods. Once a week, the participants got together at their respective GEICO facilities in ten cities across the United States. Our team showed them how to focus on quality, not quantity, using appetite-taming foods. In the process, the average person's food intake fell by more than 200 calories per day. Weight loss was easy and *occurred without hunger.*[2]

In a later study, conducted in our offices in Washington, DC, a diet change led to a similar drop in calories. The average participant lost about thirteen pounds in sixteen weeks. They did not feel hungry or deprived and were not even aware that they were eating fewer calories.[3] We have now seen the same kind of results in study after study.

This is the *appetite-taming effect* in action. Instead of needing, say, 1,800 or 2,000 calories every day to feel full, with these foods making you feel full and satisfied, you will feel ready to leave the table much sooner—perhaps hundreds of calories sooner.

The appetite-taming effect comes from a combination of factors. Among the more curious of these is something found in chili peppers. Researchers have suggested that natural compounds in peppers, called *capsaicinoids*, subtly alter taste perception so that you have less desire for fatty foods and all the calories they harbor, effectively reducing appetite.[4]

However, the most reliable appetite-taming effect is much simpler, and relates to fiber, fat, and carbohydrate. Fiber just means the roughage in fruits, vegetables, beans, and other foods from plants. Animals do not make fiber, so there is none in meat, dairy products, or eggs. A typical chili recipe, for example, is made from ground beef, which has no fiber at all. Within a few minutes of eating, the calories from beef are absorbed into your body with no fiber to slow them down. By the time you feel full, quite a few calories have come your way.

Let's say that, instead, we make our colorful Southwest Chili from black beans, green peppers, salsa, corn, lime juice, cilantro, and hot sauce. We might serve it with cornbread, or maybe on rice, with a salad, in taco shells, or just as it is. This chili has about 16 grams of fiber, which makes you feel full and satisfied with far fewer calories.

But wait, there is more. A typical meat chili serving has about 11 grams of fat, and every fat gram holds 9 calories. That is a lot. That is actually true of *any type of fat*—beef fat, chicken fat, fish fat, milk fat, and even vegetable oils. Do the math: Eleven grams of fat in the chili, multiplied by 9 calories per gram, equals 99 calories from the fat alone.

Our Southwest Chili is different. In fact, everything made from beans, grains, vegetables, and fruits is different. Beans are loaded with protein and healthy complex carbohydrate, both of which have only *4 calories per gram*—less than half the calories that are hiding in fat. So the recipe is more filling, but surprisingly low in calories.

Remember these numbers: Fat has 9 calories per gram; carbohydrate has only 4.

So while a serving of typical meat chili has about 330 calories, the bean variety has only about 240 calories, and the fiber fills you up quickly. So you'll be patting your satisfied tummy, thinking you have eaten a huge serving, but you will not have overdone it at all.

Some people might ask, *If foods are low in calories, won't we just compensate by eating more of them?* Our research has decisively shown that, with the right food choices, that does not happen. Your calorie intake will fall subtly but decisively, and you will not compensate by eating more later.

It turns out that foods high in fiber and complex carbohydrate are *appetite-tamers*. In the original research study mentioned above, we encouraged the participants to eat vegetables, fruits, beans, and whole grains, and there are endless examples of foods that emphasize these appetite-taming ingredients, as we will see in the next chapter.

A WORD ABOUT CARBOHYDRATES

A word to readers who think of bread, rice, pasta, potatoes, and other carbohydrate-rich foods as being packed with calories: These are not actually high-calorie foods at all. The fattening part is *what goes on top:* butter on bread, cheese or oil on pasta, gravy on potatoes. If you change the toppings—say, potatoes topped with grilled mushrooms, Dijon mustard, crushed black pepper, soy sauce, mint sauce, or salsa instead of fat-laden gravy, or whole-grain bread topped with jam or cinnamon instead of butter—the food is more filling with fewer calories.

Nowadays, some have tried to exonerate fatty foods and blame sugar or carbohydrates in general for weight problems. However, the benefits of cutting out fat have long been clear. In 2003, the American Dietetic Association (now the Academy of Nutrition and Dietetics) published the results of a carefully conducted research study. Overweight women were asked to eat as much as they wanted but to focus on avoiding fatty foods. They did a good job, reducing their fat intake from 33 percent of their calories to 11 percent. And, of course, low-fat foods are often high-fiber foods (fruits, vegetables, beans, and whole grains), so their fiber intake tended to climb automatically. Over the eight-month study, the average woman trimmed away 13.2 pounds (6.0 kilograms) without intentionally reducing portions at all.[5] The evidence was conclusive: Fats are by far the densest source of calories, and when we skip them, we tend to lose weight easily.[6]

Calorie-Trapping

We are off to a good start. But there are other important effects of these foods. Certain foods trap some of the calories you have ingested and carry them out with your wastes, so they cannot be absorbed. Yes, you are flushing calories down the toilet.

Tufts University researchers proved this in a particularly careful way. For a group of study volunteers, the researchers prepared everyone's foods over a six-week period. The participants came into the research center, had breakfast, and took prepared meals home with them. While some participants got whole grains (that is, with the fiber still intact, as in whole-wheat bread or brown rice), others got refined grains (with the fiber removed, as in white bread or white rice). The study focused especially on wheat, oats, and rice. Along the way, the researchers collected stool samples and measured how many calories had been "wasted"—that is, trapped in their digestive tracts and excreted, as opposed to being absorbed by the body. And the winner was...yes, whole grains. These high-fiber foods tended to carry calories out of the body with the waste.[7]

The researchers also found that the whole-grain participants got a slight boost in their metabolism. In other words, they were burning off extra calories minute by minute. Adding the number of calories carried out of the body and the extra calories burned, the whole-grain participants eliminated about 100 calories each day from that change alone—the equivalent of running a mile every morning. It adds up to a loss of more than five pounds over a year's time for an average person. This benefit is *in addition to* the weight loss that comes from adjusting other parts of your meals, as we will soon see.

Let's summarize what we have learned so far: Foods that are high in fiber and complex carbohydrate and low in fat are appetite-tamers, and certain special foods accentuate this effect. In addition, high-fiber foods trap calories. So, if we choose wisely, we get the appetite-taming effect and the calorie-trapping effect at the same time.

Calorie-Trapping

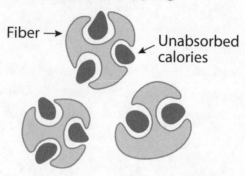

Fiber → Unabsorbed calories

So while white rice is okay, brown rice is better, because it contains calorie-trapping fiber. While white bread is okay, whole-grain bread is better, for the same reason. And remember, meat, chicken, fish, and cheese have no fiber or complex carbohydrate at all.

Metabolism-Boosting Means Burning Calories Faster

Now let's add the third breakthrough: metabolism-boosting. To explain it, let me invite you to our research center, where Liz will learn about this effect and how to put it to work.

It was four months prior to her train trip to Yale University, and Liz had not yet started the food program we were about to show her. She arrived at our offices early in the morning for preliminary tests. At our request, she had not eaten breakfast. We were about to measure her metabolism—that is, we were going to check how fast she was burning calories before she had anything to eat.

"I am sure I have a slow metabolism," Liz said. "When I was a teenager, I could eat anything, and I never gained weight. But now, I just look at food and I gain weight."

In the lobby, I introduced her to Francesca, another research volunteer who was about ten years her senior, and they began comparing notes. Francesca said that she had the same problem; she was unable to lose weight. She blamed it on her Italian heritage and her love of food. As her weight climbed, she was desperate to find a solution.

Despite very different backgrounds, the two had had remarkably similar experiences: gradual weight gain, frustration with diets, a tendency to blame themselves for diet failures, and the wish to be able to eat their favorite foods without gaining weight.

Our research technician invited Liz into the examination room and showed her to a comfortable reclining chair. He gave her a clear plastic mask to put over her mouth and nose. Feeling a bit like an astronaut, she sat still and tried to breathe normally. As the minutes went by, the researchers measured how much oxygen she inhaled and how much carbon dioxide she exhaled. With some rather simple arithmetic, the researchers used that information to calculate exactly how fast she was burning calories.

It turned out that Liz's metabolism was indeed a bit slow. Minute by minute, she was burning calories just slightly more slowly than average.

The next question was how her body would respond to food. The researchers gave her a liquid breakfast—it tasted like a vanilla milkshake. "Not so bad," Liz said. She put the mask back on, and the researchers checked her metabolism again. As the nutrients in the liquid breakfast streamed into her body, her metabolism inched upward. Although Liz did not feel anything, the research team could see the change. Her metabolism—her calorie-burning speed—kept rising. Over the next three hours, the research team checked how much oxygen her body was using and how much carbon dioxide she was exhaling. It was clear that her metabolism had increased significantly, and it remained higher for the rest of the morning.

So far, the metabolism boost was not huge, but it was a start. Our next step was to see if, over time, healthy foods would make her metabolism go higher. We would see how different foods would affect her ability to burn calories, her body weight, and her health overall.

Different Foods, Different Effects

As you eat a meal, your body uses its nutrients to power your muscles, your brain, and all the rest of you. If all goes well, your body will burn these nutrients, not store them as fat. That said, not all foods are created equal. Some give you energy; others are more likely to go to fat. Let's say we give you a spoonful of butter and then check your metabolism. What happens is...nothing. Butter did not increase your metabolism at all. Let's try two spoonfuls of butter— or three or four, or maybe half a stick of butter. You'll get sick of this pretty soon, and your metabolism just sits in neutral. Butter slides easily into your body fat without much of any calorie burn.

Now, let's try something different: a piece of ordinary whole-grain bread. It is nothing special; you could have bought it at any corner store. As you eat the bread, your calorie burn starts to rise. And your metabolism remains slightly higher than usual for a few hours.

Unlike butter, which is pure fat, whole-grain bread is rich in complex carbohydrate. Your body will break that complex carbohydrate into individual *glucose* molecules to power your muscles, light up your brain, and keep all your organs working. Those processes use up a lot of the calories. The bread is also about 20 percent protein, and it's quite a job for your body to absorb and metabolize it, so that burns calories, too.

For an average person, the after-meal calorie burn consumes about 200 calories per day. The more your foods are based on a healthful mixture of complex carbohydrate and protein, the better burn you get.

Foods That Slow Your Calorie Burn

Certain foods can hurt your metabolism. Here's how.

Inside your cells are *mitochondria*, as you might recall from high school biology. These microscopic furnaces turn the foods you eat into energy to power your body. When they are working right, you can burn through calories.

Researchers at Pennington Biomedical Research Center in Louisiana invited ten young men to join a research study in which they measured the activity of the genes that controlled their mitochondria. Then, the researchers added fatty foods to the volunteers' diets. Normally, fats make up about 30 percent of the calories in an American's diet. For the experiment, the researchers increased that to 50 percent. That is not hard to do. Chinook salmon is about 53 percent fat. A typical hot dog is in the same range. Cheese averages about 70 percent fat. Throw in some onion rings or creamy dressing on your salad, and up goes the fat content of your foods.

Three days later, the genes that control the calorie-burning mitochondria were already about 20 percent less active.[8] In other words, fatty foods slow down your "furnaces," and they do their dirty work remarkably quickly.

Fat in Cells Interferes with Calorie Burning

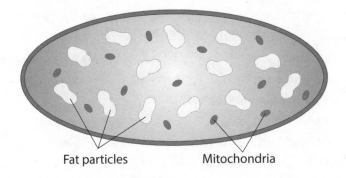

Fat particles   Mitochondria

Don't blame your body. In a way, this process makes sense. During human evolution, fatty foods were rather rare. If you were able to get your hands on fatty foods and all the dense calories they harbor, your body might want to store those calories as a hedge against a future food shortage, rather than burning them. Nowadays, storing fat is not what we are looking for. If fatty foods are chronically suppressing your metabolism, that could explain a lot.

Meanwhile, scientists at Virginia Tech found another, more disturbing, aspect of the story. Foods might actually be *poisoning* your calorie-burning ability. Here is how.

Inside your intestinal tract are millions of bacteria. Some are friendly bacteria, but others are more mischievous, producing toxic compounds. The Virginia researchers found that fatty foods make your intestinal tract more permeable to a bacterial toxin called *endotoxin*, which then slips through the intestinal wall into your bloodstream. From there, endotoxin reaches cells throughout your body, shutting down your calorie-burning ability.[9]

Some people think of fat dripping off a pork rib or butter dribbling from a corn cob onto our fingers as somehow succulent. But as it rolls down your intestinal tract, it makes it harder and harder for your cells to burn calories.

"Wait a minute," I hear you say. "Some people lose weight by *avoiding* carbohydrate and eating fatty foods like butter. How does that work?"

Not very well over the long run, as it turns out. But it is true that you could lose weight eating a pat of butter, *if that is all you ate*. A pat of butter has about 36 calories, and your body needs much more than that to meet its needs. So if you ate a pat of butter, or even a stick of butter (about 800 calories), you could lose weight, *so long as you don't eat much else*.

Low-carbohydrate fad diets promise that you will lose weight if you eat fatty foods, and avoid fruits, bread, pasta, cereals, beans, potatoes, rice, juice, and more or less everything else that has carbohydrate in it. And the net effect is that you may lose weight over the short run because you are leaving out so many foods, soon to be followed by weight gain when you get sick of being without the healthful foods you've omitted. Over the long run, you are doing no favors to your metabolism.

Special Foods for Extra Power

So far, we have seen that certain foods increase your burn after any given meal. As a rule, the best choices are fruits, vegetables, legumes, grains, and all the meals they can turn into. As you continue to eat healthful meals on a daily basis, your after-meal metabolism *gets stronger* day by day. However, certain foods have extra weight-loss power. Let me show you.

Perhaps I would like to lose weight while eating French toast. Is that possible? Actually, with a couple of tweaks, it is easy. For starters, a typical French toast recipe calls for soaking bread in eggs and whole milk, then frying it in butter. Then, on your plate, on goes more butter, plus syrup. It is easy to make the recipe milk-, egg-, and butter-free, as you will see in the recipe section. In the process, the fat content plummets. If we choose whole-grain bread, we build in appetite-taming, calorie-trapping fiber. Over time, this low-fat, high-fiber, high-complex-carbohydrate combination will boost your metabolism. So far, so good.

Now, let's think about our toppings. Blueberry syrup would add color and flavor, of course. But it might do more than that. Its color comes from natural compounds called *anthocyanins*. The name is not important; what matters is that scientists have long been studying how they affect your weight.

In a 2017 study, researchers in the United Kingdom examined pairs of female identical twins, 2,734 women in all. They found that, within each pair, the twin who ate more of certain foods tended to have less body fat, especially abdominal fat, compared with her sister.[10] At the top of the list were blueberries and other anthocyanin-rich foods. A half cup of berries each day added to breakfast cereal, tossed onto a salad, or eaten as a dessert did the trick.

At Harvard University, researchers made similar findings in the Health Professionals Follow-Up Study, the Nurses' Health Study, and the Nurses' Health Study II. Tracking the diets of 133,468 physicians and nurses, the researchers found that the more people increased their berry intake, the more weight they lost.[11] By the way, you can do the same with grapes, strawberries, or raspberries. They have anthocyanins, too, as you might have guessed from their color.

At this point, you might be wondering if a person could lose weight with a blueberry muffin or pie or a blueberry-mango salad or sorbet. The answer is yes, depending on what else goes into these foods. That is exactly what we are going to do. Our job is to put science and taste together with wonderful foods. Of course, you can also destroy their benefits by packing butter or shortening into a muffin or pie. I will show you what you need to know, and you will soon be an expert.

We are not quite done with breakfast. Imagine a small bowl of ground cinnamon. Although chefs love it for what it will do for breakfast rolls and desserts, scientists have dug into its effects on weight and blood sugar control.[12]

In a 2017 study, 116 overweight volunteers were given capsules containing raw powdered cinnamon or else placebo capsules—that is, dummy capsules with none of the spice in them—to take with their meals. The assignment to cinnamon or placebo pills was random, and the two groups were similar in age, activity, and most other characteristics. Sixteen weeks later, everyone stood on the scale. As you would expect, the placebo pills did essentially nothing. What about the participants who got the cinnamon pills? They lost almost eight pounds (3.5 kilograms) over the same period.[13]

How much cinnamon do you need to make this happen? The research team used 3 grams—about a teaspoon—per day. But you can use much less because you are using many other weight-loss foods, too. And while you could take cinnamon capsules, why not just sprinkle it onto rice pudding, your morning oatmeal, waffles, cookies, dessert nachos, apple dumplings, cake, or, yes, French toast?

Let's put a couple of slices of French toast on a plate, add a touch of cinnamon, top them with a simple blueberry syrup and sliced banana, and dig in. As you can imagine, this breakfast is delicious.

There are plenty of other power foods, and we'll cover them in the next chapter. Some are well known in other countries but new to Westerners. Some are a bit exotic. Vegetables from the sea, such as wakame, nori, and arame, are nature's original source of iodine—which your thyroid uses to keep your metabolism running strong. We can put them to work in miso soup, arame salad, and crunchy snacks. Others are as familiar as apples, pears, and strawberries.

Changes Within Your Cells

Liz was an eager pupil. She learned which foods trigger weight loss and ate them daily. Four months later, she came back to our laboratory for her final tests. It was early morning, just like the previous test. She sat in the same chair, wore the same "astronaut mask," and consumed the same vanilla-flavored shake she'd had at the beginning of the study. But while the shake gave her a calorie-burning boost at the beginning, it now gave her an even bigger boost—about 15 percent higher than before. It was clear that something had changed in her body so that she was burning calories faster after meals. She now gets that edge every day, after every meal.

After the metabolism test, Liz went to New Haven for more tests. Earlier, we left Liz in the magnetic resonance suite at Yale University. The scan took a long time. She lay patiently in the scanner as the research team looked inside her cells. The researchers then compared the results to the scan she had at the start of the study. They found that fat particles had started to dissipate from her cells and were no longer encumbering her mitochondria—her microscopic calorie burners. Her cells were transforming, so she was able to burn calories faster—more like she did as an adolescent.

On November 2, 2020, the American Medical Association published the results of this research study.[14] The food changes that Liz and the other research participants had put to work had indeed ratcheted up their metabolism. They had also improved their appetite

The After-Meal Calorie Burn

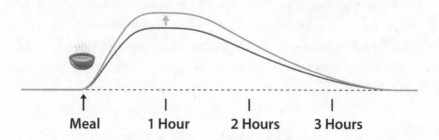

Meal	1 Hour	2 Hours	3 Hours

control. Foods with fewer calories satisfied them, and, at the same time, they were burning calories faster.

How Sweet It Is

As the research study drew to a close, the participants got together and brought in some favorite desserts to share. They had been through a lot together over the course of the study and, although they were sorry to see it coming to an end, they had much to celebrate.

Liz offered one of her favorite desserts—Black and Blue brownies (page 283).

"These are delicious," one of the other volunteers said. "And rich."

Francesca added, "You'd better hope that Dr. Barnard does not find out."

Liz smiled. "It's his recipe," she said.

Indeed, it was, and I'll tell you what's in them. First, however, let's be clear: If you had the idea that dessert cannot be healthy *and* delicious, allow me to correct that thought. In fact, if there is nothing else you get from this book, let me help you realize that you can love foods that love you back.

Don't get me wrong. Our research participants did not just eat dessert. They ate a broad array of healthful foods, and their grandmothers would have been proud of them. But the fact is that you can indeed enjoy delicious foods—including desserts—and lose weight in the process.

Okay, about those brownies. Typical recipes call for flour, butter, sugar, eggs, cocoa powder, vanilla extract, and maybe some chocolate chips. The brownies end up about 40 percent fat as a percentage of calories. That is a lot.

Liz's brownies were made with whole-wheat flour, cocoa powder, dates, blueberry fruit spread, applesauce, vanilla extract, and a secret ingredient no one suspects: a few black beans added to the batch. Sounds surprising, I know. But the "beany-ness" somehow melts away in the oven, and you are left with a brownie that is slightly richer and higher in protein. Not that you are looking for protein in a brownie, but this one is about 15 percent protein, compared with around 4 percent for the usual variety. Another big bonus: It has practically no fat at all—just 1 gram, compared to up to 18 grams for a typical brownie. With healthy complex carbohydrate and protein and so little fat, it is modest in calories and is a metabolism booster. Liz's brownies also pack 7 grams of appetite-taming fiber, compared to 1 gram for a typical recipe. Bottom line: The brownies were delicious, and they worked their metabolic magic.

Another participant, André, had brought his favorite dessert. He had combined strawberries, chunks of fresh mango, and banana slices in a clear glass bowl and sprinkled slivered almonds on top. It was simple, light, and delicious. Of course, it was a healthy choice. But then he surprised everyone with the dessert he serves friends at parties. Opening a large box, he pulled out a carrot cake with citrus cream cheese icing, and cut everyone a slice. It was soft, sweet, and filling, and no one could believe it was a healthy choice until he showed the list of ingredients. And, yes, as you will see, it is a surprisingly easy matter to modify a fattening favorite.

Of course, there are many desserts that do not love you back. But there are many that love you just fine. We will look at ways to make frozen desserts, cookies, and other sweets that, with a few simple tweaks, become metabolism boosters.

Simple Changes, Big Results

In the next chapter, we will explore the specific foods that combine the three effects you have come to know: They tame your appetite, trap calories, and boost your metabolism at the same time. As you will see, there are a great many. And they have added special effects based on natural compounds they contain. The beauty of this is that it is all free. You do not need new sneakers, barbells, or a gym membership. If you choose the right foods, weight loss is essentially automatic.

CHAPTER 2

The Best Foods for Powering Your Weight Loss

In this chapter, we will look at the edible treasures you will want to include in your routine. Each one has specific properties that will help you lose weight. Then, in the following chapter, we will look at foods that tend to cause weight gain and that you will want to avoid.

When it comes to power foods, let me encourage you to have a variety. Our goal is not to eat just one food and hope to lose a phenomenal amount of weight. Rather, each food plays its part. Let them work together.

Before we tease apart specific foods and how they work, let's imagine what a day's menu might look like.

For breakfast, how about the French toast we mentioned in chapter 1? It's light and delicious, and everyone loves it. It combines the weight-loss power of whole grains, blueberries, and cinnamon. Family members will love it, too, and will benefit as much as you do.

At lunchtime, we might start with our Very Fast Veggie Lentil Soup, along with crusty bread and a green salad with vinegar dressing. We're going for taste and heartiness, but lentils also tame your appetite and provide the full calorie-trapping effect. If you prefer, you could do the same with a black bean burrito, topped with pico de gallo.

An afternoon snack is a simple bowl of berries, mango chunks, and sliced banana, a delicate and delicious combination that draws its power from three weight-loss favorites.

At dinnertime, we'll have appetizers—a Mediterranean chickpea salad, along with grilled baby asparagus—followed by Pesto Spaghetti with Broccoli and Sun-Dried Tomatoes. Dessert could be Black and Blue Brownies or Quickie Cinnamon Rice Pudding.

By now, you can see the strategy. Each of these meals uses weight-loss ingredients, and we will discuss them in more detail in this chapter. We will not destroy their benefits by slathering them with butter and other calorie-packed toppings. We will bring out the natural taste in each food and let it work its magic. Your best friends will be fruits, vegetables, whole grains, and legumes. Certain spices and herbs are highly recommended, too. As you will see, there are a great many choices.

Of course, you may prefer to keep things simple and include convenience foods as much as possible. That's perfectly fine. The key to weight loss is to use the foods that do the work for you.

How the Research Is Done

As we have seen, Harvard researchers tracked down the foods that seem most powerful for weight loss. Here is how they did it: The Harvard team invited a large group of nurses, physicians, and other health professionals to record their food intake and then monitored their weight and overall health over many years. Among their many findings was the fact that people who emphasize certain foods in their routines tend to lose weight. For example, those who started eating more berries, broccoli, or cantaloupe ended up slimmer over time. In 2015, the Harvard team identified the following six categories of fruits and vegetables as being most strongly associated with weight loss:

1. **Berries.** Blueberries, strawberries, and their cousins.
2. **Cruciferous vegetables.** Broccoli, cauliflower, cabbage, brussels sprouts, and their relatives.
3. **Green leafy vegetables.** Spinach, chard, lettuce, and other leafy greens.
4. **Melon.** Cantaloupe and watermelon.
5. **Citrus fruits.** Oranges and grapefruit, fresh or as juice.
6. **Legumes.** Beans, peas, lentils, and products such as tofu or soy milk made from them.

These six categories are a great start; they are all healthful foods. Other researchers have added many more pieces to the puzzle. Some have brought volunteers into controlled settings where foods are prepared in precise amounts, while participants' eating habits, weight, movement, and behavior are carefully monitored. Our research team conducts studies of people living at home, eating in restaurants, and living their normal lives. The participants track their food intake and come in for laboratory testing of various kinds, and our goal is to see how foods and dietary patterns work in the real world. Other research teams do various laboratory tests, teasing apart the natural chemical compounds that make up the foods we eat. In some cases, they isolate specific compounds so we can understand how they work.

In the process, the list of weight-loss foods has grown, and we know much more about how they work. That is what you will learn in this chapter.

Let's start with spices, then work our way through the most powerful foods for weight control.

Spices

Spices do more than make foods tasty; some have specific benefits for health, including weight loss. Here are three important ones:

The Power of Cinnamon

In the previous chapter, we touched on cinnamon's weight-loss properties, which researchers have been eager to investigate.[1] As you will recall, a 2017 study showed that a teaspoon of cinnamon per day caused an average weight loss of about a half pound per week. In 2022, the *Journal of Food Biochemistry* published a meta-analysis combining the results of five prior studies, concluding that, indeed, it works.[2] And you can go easy on cinnamon if you want; it does not have to be a teaspoon every day. Keep in mind, you are not relying on cinnamon alone.

So how does it work? Scientists have isolated a natural compound that they named *cinnamaldehyde* that appears to slow down stomach emptying and increases your calorie burn. Needless to say, it is easy to use. It can top your morning oatmeal, Cream of Wheat, French toast, or pancakes and combines beautifully with bananas or other fruit. And don't forget cinnamon toast; it is great without the butter. Of course, cookies and puddings are delightful when topped with cinnamon. Some people use it as a tea, stirring a small teaspoon of ground cinnamon into hot water.

Tips for Buying and Storing Cinnamon

- Ceylon cinnamon (*Cinnamomum verum*), sometimes called true cinnamon, is what you want. More common in the United States are Chinese (*Cinnamomum cassia*), Indonesian (or Korintje, *Cinnamomum burmannii*), and Saigon (*Cinnamomum loureiroi*) cinnamon (also called Vietnamese cinnamon). These latter three are referred to as *cassia*, and all have more bang than the more well-behaved Ceylon cinnamon, but they also contain coumarin, which can be harmful to the liver (Ceylon cinnamon contains only small traces of coumarin). You can see the difference: In cross section, a true cinnamon stick is round, but a cassia stick curls in from both sides, like a scroll.

- Store cinnamon in an airtight container to keep out moisture, and keep it in a dark, dry, cool place.
- Powdered cinnamon will start losing its potency a year or so after opening. Stick cinnamon lasts longer.
- Organic cinnamon is widely available and worth it.

The Power of Hot Peppers

Because chili peppers can burn your tongue, many people have wondered if they might help us burn off unwanted weight. That fiery sensation comes from a natural compound called *capsaicin*, one of a group of compounds called *capsaicinoids*, as we learned earlier. Peppers also contain less-hot compounds, called *capsinoids*. Apart from its role in spicy foods, capsaicin is also mixed into creams for sore joints; after the tingling stops, joint pain is less severe.

Researchers have learned a great deal about all these compounds. First of all, capsaicinoids may help tame the appetite. Specifically, they appear to alter taste perception so that you are less drawn to fatty foods and prefer carbohydrates, which have fewer calories.[3]

More important, researchers have examined their effects on calorie-burning. The studies themselves are surprising. Researchers measured body temperature on the forehead, neck, and eardrum. Within minutes of eating a hot pepper, body temperature rose, meaning that the body was releasing calories as body heat. It stayed higher than normal for more than an hour. Researchers also measured how much oxygen the body was using up and how much carbon dioxide was being exhaled minute by minute, which indicated the body's metabolism speed. These measures, too, were boosted by compounds in peppers.

In a 2009 study, eighty overweight people were given capsules containing either capsinoids or a placebo. Over the next twelve weeks, the capsinoid group had an uptick in metabolism and lost abdominal fat.[4] Other researchers have found the same thing, and some evidence suggests a stronger effect in individuals who are more overweight, compared with thinner individuals.[5]

All of this raises an obvious question: Not everyone wants a singed tongue, so would ordinary bell peppers work? Unfortunately no. Researchers compared hot capsaicin-rich Cayenne Long Slim peppers against California Wonder bell peppers, which are not hot at all. The hot peppers boost metabolism; the non-hot ones do not. What really seems to matter is the amount of capsaicin or related compounds in the pepper. Typical bell peppers have none. They add crunch to a salad but will not boost your metabolism.

Some research teams are developing varieties that are not hot but contain capsinoids with some metabolism-boosting ability,[6] and some manufactureres have made extracts for sale as nutritional supplements. They are not widely available, and the safety of their extraction and manufacturing processes is not clear. So the best answer appears to be to stick with food sources, not extracts.

Peppers make black beans, bean burritos, and other healthful dishes come alive and make these healthful foods irresistible. Unlike other toppings, such as shredded cheese or bacon bits, peppers are free of fat and cholesterol. Even so, the weight-loss benefits may be modest and easily overwhelmed when an innocent hot pepper is crammed with pork and cheese.

HOT, HOT, HOT—OR NOT

An ordinary bell pepper is not hot at all. Banana peppers, pepperoncini, and poblano (or ancho) peppers are slightly spicier. Jalapeños are a noticeable step up. Beyond them are cayenne, tabasco, habanero, and ghost peppers (check your life insurance policy). If you grow peppers, harvest them early to keep them tame, or leave them on the vine longer to build the heat.

Although we find peppers in Indian curries, Italian arrabbiata sauce, sriracha sauce in Thailand, and dishes from China to North Africa, their original home was Latin America. It was Christopher Columbus who began their worldwide distribution.

In 1912, a Parke-Davis pharmacist named Wilbur Scoville came up with a way to quantify peppers' "heat." Feeding small amounts to volunteers, he gradually diluted the pepper more and more until the heat was no longer detectable. The amount of dilution gave each pepper a number on what came to be called the Scoville scale. Today, the capsaicinoid content of peppers is measured directly using sophisticated laboratory methods.

The Power of Ginger

Ginger is delicious, of course. Many people have speculated about its health benefits. By 2019, fourteen different weight-loss studies had been completed and were summarized in a meta-analysis. The verdict was that ginger does indeed cause weight loss—specifically, loss of belly fat.[7] Whether that is because of a specific effect of ginger on abdominal fat or because abdominal fat is the first to go when you are losing weight is not clear.

Scientists have isolated ginger's biologically active compound and named it *gingerol*. It is a relative of capsaicin (the "hot" in hot peppers, as we saw above), but is more tangy than hot, and it exists in several related forms. Cooking mellows ginger's flavor, but when dried, it produces natural compounds called *shogaols* (from the Japanese word for ginger, *shōga*) with about twice the zip found in gingerol.

Apart from a direct effect on body weight, it makes vegetables taste great, so it guides us toward healthful foods. For example, carrot and ginger soup is delicious and colorful, especially topped with a bit of parsley. You'll probably not even think about the gingerol or beta-carotene (see below) inside, but there they are.

Japanese ginger dressing turns a simple salad into a delight. Of course, there are ginger tea, gingerbread, and ginger cookies. And ginger is equally at home on stir-fried vegetables (e.g., bok choy), fried rice, grilled tofu, and the cucumber roll proudly presented by any sushi chef.

Tips for Buying and Storing Ginger

- Both fresh ginger root and ground ginger are fine to use. In a recipe, one tablespoon of fresh ginger is equivalent to one half teaspoon of ground ginger. Be aware that ginger's taste may intensify over time in a dish, so you might go easy.
- Ginger root should be firm, with no soft spots.
- Choose a root with thin skin that easily comes off with your fingernail. Thick, tough skin is a sign of an old, dried-out root.
- Ginger will keep for a week or so at room temperature. Unpeeled, in a sealed plastic bag in the refrigerator, it will last for weeks. Frozen, it will last for months.
- When you are ready to peel it, scrape off the skin with a teaspoon.
- If you are flavoring a soup or stew, cut ginger into coin-sized chunks, which can be easily retrieved to control the spiciness, unlike grated or ground ginger. For other uses, grated or ground is fine.
- In the Asian section of grocery stores, you will find pickled ginger, ready for use.

In the recipe section, explore the dishes using cinnamon, peppers, and ginger, and think about ways you might incorporate them into your routine.

Shauné

Shauné grew up in Kansas City, Missouri. There was plenty of tasty, but not entirely healthful, food at home: sloppy joes, meat loaf, fried chicken, fried egg and bologna sandwiches, hot dogs, and vegetables seasoned with fatback, ham hocks, or bacon. On Sundays or holidays after church, the family often frequented all-you-can-eat buffets.

As a child, Shauné found herself gaining weight. She was very active, getting plenty of outside exercise, "but you cannot out-exercise a bad diet," she said. As her weight increased, her self-confidence suffered.

Her mother was in a weight-loss program, and at age twelve, Shauné joined her. Together, they went on a weight roller coaster, going up and down and never reaching their goals. For Shauné, diets were a struggle. Restricting portions and tracking her servings of this or that food group was not easy for a child, and she did not really understand which foods were good for her.

Over the years, she tried many different diets—cabbage soup, low-calorie diets, and everything else. Sometimes her appetite rebelled, leading to binges, regrets, and shame. Her doctor prescribed the appetite suppressant phentermine, which made her heart race and left her feeling jittery.

At twenty-seven, she married. Anticipating the wedding day, she hoped to be able to wear her mother's wedding dress, which was far smaller than she was. She restricted her calories and exercised as much as she could and succeeded in losing fifty pounds. But after the wedding, she and her husband settled into married life, and the lost weight came back, and then some.

She had been working as a journalist for a major Washington, DC, newspaper and eventually decided to leave and start her own business. But that meant working practically around the clock to succeed and neglecting her health in the process. Eventually, she reached 278 pounds. Something had to change.

The solution presented itself in an unusual way. Shauné and a friend started walking together on a regular basis. In the Maryland woods, she connected with nature. Sometimes, she would stop and listen to the birds and to the breeze rustling the trees. She started to take stock of what she wanted in her life.

She happened upon a recipe book for green smoothies. It sounded healthy, and she decided to try it. She put kale, spinach, cucumbers, frozen strawberries, mangoes, cherries, and flaxseeds into a blender along with a couple of cups of water, and she loved the refreshing taste. On weekends, she bagged up the ingredients and kept them in the freezer, ready to blend during the week.

She noticed that she was losing weight without really trying. This was unexpected and exciting. She found a health coach who helped her explore more food options: "My world opened up to all the things that I could eat, and I was able to break out of the restrictions I had lived with so long."

She read a book called *The China Study*, by T. Colin Campbell and Thomas M. Campbell II, which talked about the relationship between foods and health. And now, there was no turning back. She dumped dieting for good and focused on healthy foods. She sprinkled ginger and chili powder onto lentils and chickpeas, along with garlic, mustard, fennel, onion, cumin, cardamon, turmeric, and black pepper to make a fragrant and flavorful dal, and found that it got even better when she saved some for the next day.

Gradually, she lost one hundred pounds. Her doctor was impressed by her amazing weight loss and the improvements in her blood pressure, cholesterol, and blood sugar. Today, she feels free from the restrictions she had for so long, and she loves her exploration of healthful foods and new flavors.

She decided she had to spread this information to others. She became a Food for Life instructor with the Physicians Committee for Responsible Medicine and launched TheShaunéLife.com to provide health coaching and cooking classes. Soon, her mother joined her classes. Together, they tweak the recipes she grew up with.

What brings us back to health? "Our power is on the end of the fork," she says.

Fruits

The Power of Blueberries and Their Friends

In the previous chapter, we bragged about blueberries, and for good reason. When Harvard University researchers tracked the fruits associated with weight loss, these little berries were at the top of the list, and British researchers found much the same thing.[8]

Their majestically colored anthocyanins are natural antioxidants that have also been studied for their effects on memory. University of Cincinnati researchers found memory-boosting effects of blueberry juice in older people who had been troubled by memory lapses. The amount that seemed to do the trick was two cups of juice per day for three months.[9] Concord grape juice did the same thing.[10] Later researchers have jumped in and reported benefits for both short- and long-term memory in what has become an active area of brain research.[11]

However, it may well be that berries' weight-loss benefits mainly come from their nutrient makeup—that is, from the fact that they are rich in healthful carbohydrate and appetite-taming fiber, with very little fat and few calories. A full cup of blueberries has only about one third the calories in a typical twenty-ounce soda.

In the kitchen, they can top your morning cornflakes, oatmeal, pancakes, or French toast. They are eager to jump into pancake batter, muffin mix, and smoothies. At lunchtime, they bring a delightful tartness to salads and add flavor and color to banana bread, and, of course, jams and jellies. As desserts, they become pies, tarts, cobblers, and blueberry "nice cream"—that is, dairy-free ice cream. Or combine with sliced mango and banana. I listed it above as a snack, but it is a delightful dessert with no regrets.

Have a look at the recipe section and see what calls to you. Or just pick up some berries and include them in your routine.

Tips for Buying and Storing Blueberries

- Berries should be plump and deep blue.
- Buying organic is a good idea. Pesticides are often used on conventional varieties.
- Resist the urge to wash them until just before using them. Surface moisture can lead to mold.
- Store berries in the refrigerator, not on the countertop.
- Frozen berries are convenient, economical, and have a long freezer life.
- It pays not to undo their benefits with unhealthful additions. A blueberry muffin or tart prepared properly is part of a weight-loss solution. But pack in the butter, shortening, and so on, and the benefits are lost.

Anthocyanins are also found in blackberries, strawberries, raspberries, cherries, grapes, and many other berries, as well as in autumn leaves as they show their beautiful colors. Don't eat the leaves. The rest can all be part of your weight-loss menu.

"Can berries really help me lose weight?" you may ask. Not if they are just sitting on the store shelves looking pretty. Most people neglect them completely. Bring some home, build them into your routine, and you will see.

The Power of Apples and Pears

The Harvard team found that apples and pears were also strongly associated with weight loss. These everyday foods are rich in fiber, which has almost no calories. They also hold water, which has exactly no calories. No fat, plenty of metabolism-boosting healthful carbohydrate—they are made for weight loss. So, an apple a day really does keep the pounds away.

Now, wait a minute. Apples have natural sugars, which is why they are so sweet. You might ask, "Won't they cause weight gain? What if we overdo it on apples or other fruit? Won't we gain weight?"

Brazilian researchers tested that question in a rather extreme way. In a research study, they invited women, all between thirty and fifty years old, to eat apples every day. But to make it a real test, the participants were asked to eat *three* apples every day, day after day. A second group was asked to have three pears every day.

During the ten-week study, the women filled up on more fruit than anyone could imagine eating—210 apples or pears per person. But because apples and pears are high in fiber and full of water, women in both fruit groups actually found themselves eating *fewer* calories every day despite the seemingly large amount of food they were eating. Let me make this clear: By *adding* apples and pears, they were taking in *fewer* calories than before. Apples and pears crowd out higher-calorie foods. In a word, adding fruit subtracts calories overall, strange as that may sound. And, you guessed it, they lost weight.[12]

Of course, the point is not to eat three apples or three pears a day—although you could if you wanted to. The point is to include these healthful weight-loss foods—hopefully in a generous variety—in your routine.

Dried Fruit Is Slimming, Too

What about dried fruit? Some people fear that drying fruit concentrates its natural sugars and turns a slimming food into a fattening food. This idea was put to the test by a team of Florida researchers. They asked a group of healthy women to have about three ounces (75 grams) of dried apple each day. Although most people tend to gradually gain weight year by year, the opposite happened for these women. After a year, they had lost more than three pounds (1.5 kilograms) on average.[13] Not huge, but that is the weight loss associated with the dried apples alone, without cutting calories, adding exercise, or making any other diet changes at all. In other words, dried fruit is okay and even helpful. Apple juice appears to be weight-neutral.[14]

Apples and pears are natural appetite-tamers and are enormously versatile. Starting your day, they can be eaten as is, sliced to top your morning cereal, or added to a fruit salad. After dinner, they become apple pie, applesauce, apple crisp, and apple cobbler (don't forget the cinnamon), and here again they play well with berries or other fruit ingredients. At holiday parties, they are part of stuffing and used for candied apples. If you are celebrating, the traditional apple brandy from northern France, called calvados, goes perfectly with an apple tart.

A quick reminder: These healthful foods can easily become fattening foods by packing butter, shortening, or oils into the recipes.

The key is to take advantage of the healthful ingredients without adding the problem ingredients.

Tips for Buying and Storing Apples and Pears

- Have fun trying different varieties, if you have not done so already: Gala, Red Delicious, Fuji, Honeycrisp, and McIntosh apples; Bartlett, Anjou, and Bosc pears, among others. Whether you like them screamingly sweet or more subtle, they all work. See which ones you like best.
- Check the color. A bright red color is a sign that an apple has soaked up plenty of sunshine in the growing process and will be nice and sweet (of course, Golden Delicious apples are naturally golden, and Granny Smiths are green; don't hold that against them).
- Apples should be firm; a soft apple is overripe.
- A ripe pear is mostly firm, too. But press gently near the stem end; if it has a little give, it's ripe.
- This is one place where buying organic is a really good idea. If you were eating a banana or an orange, you would throw away the peel along with any chemicals lurking on the surface. When you eat an apple or a pear, you eat the peel, too. So organic is best.
- When you get home, wash them so they will be ready when you are.
- Apples like to be stored at cool temperatures. They also like humidity—for example, being covered with a damp paper towel.
- Pears ripen at room temperature. You can slow that process down, if you like, by putting them in the refrigerator.
- To prevent browning of leftover sliced apples, place them in water for thirty minutes with a bit of salt. Then drain and store in the refrigerator.

The Power of Mangoes and Papayas

Mangoes and papayas are like long-lost cousins. Mangoes arose in the Indian subcontinent, while papayas are from Mexico and Central America, but in the kitchen, they have a lot in common. Like nearly all fruit, they are very low in fat and high in appetite-taming fiber and healthful carbohydrate to boost your after-meal metabolism. Despite their sweetness, mangoes and papayas have a surprisingly low glycemic index, meaning that their natural sugars enter your body gradually, giving you energy without spiking your blood sugar.

Both fruits get their yellow-orange color from *beta-carotene*, the natural antioxidant also found in carrots and sweet potatoes. Although beta-carotene is known for its cancer-prevention role, it has also been studied for its role in blocking weight gain.[15]

For starters, scientists found that people with more beta-carotene circulating in their blood tend to be slimmer and healthier than those with lower levels of beta-carotene.[16] At first scientists suggested that the reason overweight people have so little beta-carotene in their blood is that their fat cells soak up the beta-carotene in their bodies, leaving very little to circulate in their blood. However, a 2017 study found that beta-carotene does indeed encourage weight loss. Researchers in Jacksonville, Florida, recruited overweight children, ages eight to eleven, and taught them and their families about healthier diets and exercise. At the same time, the researchers gave half the children capsules containing beta-carotene and related compounds. The other half received placebos that looked like the real thing but contained no active compounds. After six months, the researchers carefully measured the fat around the children's organs and under their skin using magnetic resonance imaging (MRI). It turned out that the children receiving the beta-carotene supplements were slimmer, with less body fat than the other children.[17]

If these fruits are new to you, just taste them and it will be love at first bite. Starting at breakfast, they are fresh and delicious as is. At lunch, they combine beautifully with strawberries, raspberries, blackberries, and kiwis as a fruit salad. Top with lime or mint leaves. For a refreshing drink, add mangoes to tea, lemonade, or water. To make a fun salsa, add mango chunks to hot peppers. Mangoes and papayas go great in smoothies and frozen desserts.

How to Cut a Mango

You can always buy a mango slicer, but you can open a mango in thirty seconds with nothing but a sharp knife and a drinking glass.

On a cutting board, stand the mango on one end. Slice downward, slightly off-center, gliding along one side of the pit. Do the same on the other side. You now have two halves of the mango, plus the central section holding the pit. Then, using an ordinary drinking glass, take one of the mango halves and pass it onto the edge of the glass so that the peel goes outside the glass and the pulp plops inside. Do the same with the other half. Slice and serve.

How to Cut a Papaya

The quick and easy way to eat a papaya is to slice it in two lengthwise, scoop out the seeds, and serve it like a boat with a spoon.

If you are serving guests, you'll want a bit more elegance. Just cut the papaya in two lengthwise, scoop out the seeds, and then slice away the peel, as if you are giving your papaya a rather coarse shave with your knife. Finally, lay the papaya on your cutting board and cut it crosswise into slices. Serve with lime wedges.

Tips for Buying and Storing Mangoes and Papayas

- Small yellow mangoes are delicious, consistent, and free of fibrous strands.

- A hard, green mango is not ripe. Leave it at room temperature (not in the refrigerator) until it is soft and yellow or red. To hasten the ripening process, you can use the famous bag trick that works for bananas (see below).
- Canned mangoes are convenient and have the same benefits as fresh mangoes.
- Papayas should be purchased ripe or nearly ripe, yellow, and fragrant. That is no easy task if you are at a distance from where they are grown. If you are buying a green papaya, I suggest also buying a copy of Samuel Beckett's *Waiting for Godot*.

The Power of Bananas

Bananas are more substantial than most other fruits. They satisfy the appetite with surprisingly few calories and contribute to a significant after-meal metabolism boost. As an afternoon snack, they cannot be beat. Let's say you are at a convenience store looking at the banana display and the rack of candy bars. Let's compare.

A Snickers bar weighs about two ounces. The label lists 250 calories, and nearly half of those calories come from fat (cocoa butter, milk fat, and palm oil) that is itching to add to your body fat. Some of those fat particles will jump into your muscle and liver cells, interfere with your mitochondria, and set you up for continued weight gain. Even worse, much of that fat is *saturated* fat—that is, "bad" fat that can raise your cholesterol level and is linked to Alzheimer's disease.[18] Who needs it?

A banana is different. It is filling like a candy bar but has fewer than half the calories (about 115, for an average banana). The banana has almost no fat. Instead, it provides a modest amount of protein, plus a healthy mixture of natural sugars and starches with a low glycemic index. After any sort of athletic endeavor, a banana is perfect for rebuilding the glycogen (stored energy) in your liver and muscles to recharge your batteries.

At the breakfast table, bananas can top your breakfast cereal, be added to pancakes, waffles, or muffins, or be eaten as is. They work beautifully in a fruit salad, in banana bread, or just peeled and eaten as a snack.

Above, I mentioned "nice cream" made with berries. Integral to it are frozen bananas blended with a nondairy milk (for example, soy milk, oat, pistachio, hazelnut, or almond milk). It has zero cholesterol, almost no fat, and is light and delicious.

If you couldn't get the idea of a Snickers bar out of your mind, here's chocolate done one step better: Make a chocobananasicle by cutting peeled bananas in half crosswise and inserting a popsicle stick into each half. Dip in melted dark chocolate and freeze on a baking sheet. Yummy and healthy!

How about a banana split? In the recipe section, you'll see how to do it right. It is super-easy and really impressive.

Tips for Buying and Storing Bananas

- Although buying organic is always a good idea, conventionally grown bananas will not deliver much in the way of pesticide residues, because the peel is discarded.
- If you buy green bananas, leave them at room temperature (not in the refrigerator) to allow them to ripen. The warmer the spot, the sooner they will ripen.
- If you are feeling impatient, put green bananas in a paper bag and close it up. This traps the natural ethylene coming from the bananas and speeds the ripening process. Adding an already ripe banana or apple to the bag will help.
- Bananas are sweetest when fully yellow with a few freckles.
- To freeze ripe bananas for future use in smoothies, bread, or muffins, just peel them, put them in a freezer-safe container or bag, and mark the date on the outside. Before freezing, you may wish to slice the bananas, put them on a baking sheet or

waxed paper, and freeze for two hours. Then put them in a bag for long-term freezing. That way, you can easily measure out the amount you need.

Other Fruits

There are, of course, countless other fruits. Oranges, plums, peaches, cherries, and all the other delights help control the appetite and give you a metabolic edge.

There are, however, two fruits that will stall your weight loss. Avocados are delicious, but, unlike their botanical cousins, they get about 80 percent of their calories from fat. That is huge. Luckily, most of the fat is *monounsaturated* fat, which is better for your heart than *saturated* fat (the "bad" fat that raises cholesterol). Even so, all types of fat—even "good" fats—contribute equally to body fat. If you are trying to shed some weight, I suggest setting them aside for now.

Coconuts are not only high in fat, they are high in *saturated* fat.[19] Same for palm oil.[20] Despite the efforts of food manufacturers to advance the myth that coconut and palm oils are somehow healthy, I would encourage you to avoid them *completely*. Ditto for coconut milk.

Falling in Love with Fruit

If fruit is not yet your thing, start by buying a few you think you might like and just keep them around—in your kitchen, at your desk, or in another handy place. Bananas, Fuji apples, or a bowl of mandarin oranges. Maybe some cherries, dates, or a little dish of raisins. Sooner or later, they will call your name, and you'll discover how good they are. And your friends will appreciate your generosity, because fresh fruit is the ultimate shareable food.

If you bought a bit too much, don't worry. The key for now is to have fruit in your life, so that you will turn to it when hunger arrives.

POWER FOODS FOR WEIGHT LOSS

The following foods and ingredients have been shown in research studies to support weight loss. Note that some categories overlap. Broccoli, for example, is both a green vegetable and a cruciferous vegetable.

Spices

Cinnamon

Hot peppers

Ginger

Fruits

Berries: blueberries, strawberries, raspberries, blackberries, etc.

Apples

Pears

Dried fruit: raisins, dried apples, apricots, etc.

Mangoes

Papayas

Squash

Bananas

Other fruit: oranges, plums, peaches, cherries, etc., but not
    avocados or coconuts

Beans, Peas, and Lentils

Beans: black beans, pinto beans, chickpeas, etc.

Peas

Lentils

Soybeans and soy products: tofu, tempeh, miso, soy-based
    meat analogues

Whole Grains

Oats

Corn

Brown rice

Other grains: millet, wheat, amaranth, etc.

Pasta

Vegetables

Green vegetables: spinach, Swiss chard, asparagus,
watercress, lettuce, etc.

Cruciferous vegetables: broccoli, cauliflower, brussels
sprouts, kale, cabbage, collards

Orange vegetables: sweet potatoes, carrots

Starchy vegetables: potatoes, but not fried potatoes
(French fries, potato chips)

Sea Vegetables

Nori

Wakame

Arame

The Power of Beans and Their Cousins

There is nothing cuter than a bean flower. Eating a plate of black
beans, you would never imagine how the plant started out, emerging
timidly from the soil, then modestly unveiling its blossoms, like little
purple jewels. Its many cousins are jewels, too, both in the garden
and in the kitchen.

Black beans are native to the Americas and turn into soup, tacos,
and nachos. Chickpeas are originally Turkish, botanists tell us, and
are now everywhere and wonderfully versatile. They become hummus, falafel, and curries, and turn a salad into a meal. Lentils are
of Middle Eastern origin and become soups, salads, dal, papadums,
and burgers. In East Asia, soybeans are king. They are so versatile,
they turn into edamame, soy milk, tofu, tempeh, miso, and plant-
based versions of everything from bacon and sausage to fish fillets

and burgers. One day someone will figure out how to turn soybeans into snow tires and lawn furniture.

This is the legume family—beans, peas, and lentils, and all the things they become. Compared with fruit, they are much higher in protein. They are also rich in calcium, iron, and appetite-taming, calorie-trapping fiber. They have basically no fat for you to store and provide a perfect combination of complex carbohydrate and protein for a good after-meal burn.

Their appetite-taming effect, in particular, has attracted scientific attention. Researchers have found that including beans or their legume cousins in a meal will lead you to stop eating before you've overdone it[21] and will lead to significant weight loss.[22] So, at a restaurant, if you choose bean chili over meat chili or have a bean burrito instead of a meat burrito, the bean variety is a weight-loss winner every time.

THE MIGHTY BEAN

One of our research participants brought her husband to a research meeting so he could sit in on the discussion and pick up a few tips. He had health issues of his own—he was seriously overweight and had a long-standing cholesterol problem. His wife was concerned that he would follow in the footsteps of his father, who had succumbed to a heart attack in his early fifties. The group agreed to let him sit in every week.

While his wife was losing weight on the regimen we were testing and her tastes gravitated to lighter dishes—rice, vegetables, and fruits—for him, it was a different story. A meal was not a meal if meat was not at the center of the plate. "I suppose that's why I'm heavy," he said. "But I love food, and a meal ought to have substance."

What helped him, surprisingly enough, turned out to be beans. He loved tacos, so he tried filling them with pureed pinto

beans or black beans instead of meat, along with the usual lettuce, salsa, and hot peppers, and they worked out great. From
there, he tried burritos, chili, and various casseroles, and he
found he was getting the "substance" he was looking for.
Needless to say, his fiber intake went up and calories went
down, even though his meals were filling and satisfying.

As it turned out, he began dropping pounds even more
rapidly than his wife had been. She was happy for them both
and hoped to be able to keep him around a bit longer.

Here's the problem: Beans have been forgotten. Although our
grandparents knew all about beans and found them satisfying and
inexpensive, nowadays they have taken a back seat to meaty fare. It's
good to remember a few favorites.

Crack open a can of black bean soup. Serve it with rice, toast, or
a baked potato, and add a salad or green vegetable.

Black beans and pinto beans work beautifully in dips, burritos,
or tacos or just as is, with a bit of pico de gallo, also called *salsa
Mexicana*, the simple topping made from freshly diced tomatoes,
onions, jalapeños, cilantro, and lime juice.

Broad beans or limas can be mashed with garlic and salt and
used in place of mashed potatoes to top off casseroles and shepherd's
pie for a change of pace.

Lentil soup is in every grocery store; choose the vegetarian brands.
And it is easy to make on your stovetop, flavored with garlic, cumin,
curry powder, thyme, pepper, lemon juice, and the like. Dal is a traditional Indian staple. It is extremely nutritious, served with rice.

As we saw earlier, beans can even be used in brownies, making
them more substantial, not to mention healthier. Sounds strange,
but it works.

If you are new to beans, canned beans are convenient and inexpensive. But cooking from scratch is really easy. If you are fearful of the

time involved, remember that you do not actually have to supervise the process. Just soak them overnight, change the water, bring to a boil, then cover and simmer for sixty to ninety minutes, or however long it takes for them to become soft. Always be sure to cook them well.

Beans do not need lard, butter, ground beef, or other greasy additives, but that has not stopped people from throwing these unhealthy ingredients into the pot. Some Mexican restaurants mistakenly maintain that lard is "traditional" in beans. It is anything but. Beans have been grown in Latin America for millennia. It was not until the Spanish arrived with pigs that lard went into the beans.

The Physicians Committee for Responsible Medicine recently surveyed Mexican restaurants and found that, while lard is still commonly used in Texas and New Mexico, it is fading fast in California, and has been mostly tossed out of Washington, DC. Correspondingly, among Latino populations, obesity is much less common where lard is not used.

Beans can be elegant. At the Equinox restaurant, just down the block from the White House in Washington, DC, legendary chef Todd Gray serves truffled white bean soup, flavored with cipollini onions, fingerling potatoes, and winter black truffle. Accompany it with butter lettuce and radicchio salad with Cara Cara oranges, flavored with English cucumber, candied pecans, and pickled fennel, and follow it with sesame-glazed eggplant and crispy tofu, with sweet peppers, vidalia onions, and cucumber-papaya slaw.

Beans can also be very basic. Many years ago, I happened to be in Brighton, on England's southern coast, and, through a chip shop's plate-glass window, I could see people squirting vinegar on French fries—a rather novel idea, I thought. But the strangest thing was a scoop of neon-green something or other topping the fries. I went inside to see what was being served.

After first teaching me not to use the term "French fries" for what are obviously *English chips*, the server then introduced me to mushy peas. Larger than typical garden peas, they are left a bit longer in the field before harvest. I tried them, vinegar and all, and they were indeed delicious.

THE SECRET TO DIGESTIBILITY

Some newcomers to the bean aisle fear that beans might cause gassiness. Here is a tip: Start small. Some people who resolve to eat better try to replace a sixteen-ounce steak with sixteen ounces of beans. That is too much. The steak had no fiber at all; in fact, it can be constipating. Beans are among the highest-fiber foods you can find. If your natural digestive bacteria (your gut microbiome) have not met beans before, they might get a bit ornery with this newcomer. So have a small portion. *A little bit goes a long way,* and your digestive tract will soon adapt. Be sure the beans are well cooked. That means *soft*. There are no al dente beans.

Chickpeas are especially handy. With a touch of dressing and some minced celery and garlic, they make a lovely starter. Combined with other beans, they become a three- or four-bean salad.

Hummus, a Middle Eastern staple, has become widely popular. Although all grocery stores carry it, you can make your own in a food processor in five minutes. It will be tastier and healthier, and you can adjust the creaminess by adding extra water. There's no need for oil at all.

Chickpeas are also used in curries and, of course, in falafel. Chickpeas also transform into a thin unleavened pancake, called *farinata* in Italy or *socca* in Nice. Sprinkled with pepper, it is as addicting as it is simple.

Soybeans are in a class by themselves. They have somewhat more fat than other beans but were found by Harvard researchers to be strongly associated with weight loss—more so than most other foods, surprisingly enough. That is, people who increase their intake of soy foods tend to be slimmer as the years go by.

SOY POWER

In addition to their apparent weight-loss benefits, soybeans have a cholesterol-lowering effect over and above what would be expected by the fact that they have no cholesterol or animal fat.[23] And contrary to common mythology, women who consume soy milk, tofu, tempeh, miso soup, or other soy products regularly have about 30 percent *lower* risk of developing breast cancer, compared with women who consume little or no soy products.[24] For women previously diagnosed with breast cancer, soy products are associated with better survival.[25] The credit appears to go to *isoflavones,* natural compounds that have favorable effects on hormonal conditions.

Menopausal women can reduce the frequency of troubling hot flashes by nearly 90 percent with a combination of a plant-based diet, minimizing fats, and including one half cup of soybeans in their routine each day.[26] The key is to use *whole* soybeans (soy milk and tofu are healthy, of course, but are not as isoflavone-rich), and to avoid animal products and oily foods completely. Start with non-GMO soybeans (available online), pressure-cook them for forty minutes, then separate them into half-cup servings. Use them like pine nuts on salads or in soups. For extra credit, spread the pressure-cooked soybeans out on a parchment-covered baking sheet and bake for an hour at 350 degrees Fahrenheit. Season with salt, cayenne, garlic powder, basil, oregano, and the like. You can also buy roasted soybeans (e.g., Laura brand Tosteds).

P. F. Chang's restaurants introduced many diners to tofu with their signature *lettuce wrap*. Strands of sautéed tofu, chopped mushrooms and water chestnuts, rice wine vinegar, hoisin sauce, and soy sauce are wrapped in a butter lettuce leaf, and you just pop it into your mouth like a taco.

If you are new to tofu, you will find that it has really no flavor on its own, very much like an egg white. But it takes on the flavors you add, from Szechuan and sweet and sour sauces, to the soy sauce and dill you marinate it in, to the cherries that make cherry cheesecake. Because it is so versatile, cooks soon become enamored with it and find ways to turn it into puddings, scrambles, burgers, ricotta, cottage cheese, and lots of other marvels.

If you're trying tofu for the first time, you might try some smoked or baked tofu (you'll find it refrigerated at most grocery stores). Cut it up on a salad or pop it in a stir-fry with vegetables. Or go to any reputable Chinese restaurant (especially Szechuan or Hunan) and choose one of the tofu (bean curd) dishes, like ma po tofu (without the pork). For this experiment, fried varieties are especially tasty, although you'll soon gravitate to the non-fried versions. Have the tofu in a flavorful, low-oil sauce with vegetables and rice, and see what you think.

CAN TOFU PROMOTE MENTAL HEALTH?

Some people who are on the moody side get a noticeable mood-balancing effect from starting their day with tofu or tempeh. This seems to be particularly true for those whose breakfasts are typically loaded with fruit or bread—which are a bit light on protein; scientists have suggested that such an overly light meal may elevate serotonin levels in the brain, leading to a feeling of sluggishness or moodiness. Tofu and tempeh have the opposite effect. They are high in healthful protein, which blocks serotonin production, while also being free of the cholesterol and animal fat found in bacon and sausage.

If you are feeling chronically moody or depressed, or if you are a woman who feels particularly out of sorts at *that* time of the month, try the recipes for grilled tofu or tempeh in the recipe section. Both cook up quickly and store easily for later in the week. They may just give your day the start it needs.

Just Amazing

Our legume friends have lent themselves to all sorts of other creative uses. I recently gave a lecture at a large Florida hospital, and afterward, the hospital chef offered a breakfast buffet including two pans of scrambled eggs. One had plain eggs; the other was adorned with red and green peppers. There was toast and fresh fruit on the side. Everything was delicious, and the assembled physicians gobbled them up.

The chef then explained that there were actually no eggs on the buffet at all. He had used a product called Just Egg. It turns out that mung beans—the kind that are often sprouted and used for salads and in Asian dishes—have a protein that can transform into a product that is virtually indistinguishable from scrambled eggs. Who'd have thought it? You won't know the difference until you look at your cholesterol test. Look for it in the refrigerator case. Just Egg pours into your frying pan, just like a beaten egg (minus the cholesterol), ready to scramble.

Tips for Buying and Storing Legumes

- Dried beans, peas, and lentils are very economical. For extra savings, you can find them in the bulk aisle at about half the price of those sold prepackaged.

- Organically grown beans are widely available at health food stores and online.
- Canned beans are convenient and perfectly healthful. Salt-free versions are available.
- When buying tofu, soy milk, or other soy products, choose organic. By US law, organic foods cannot be genetically modified.
- Tofu comes in a variety of textures, from extra firm to extra soft. For grilling, firmer is better. Silken tofu is great for making sauces, smoothies, puddings, and dips.
- Some tofu brands are boxed and shelf-stable for long periods.
- Many tofu brands are especially good sources of calcium, as you will see on the label.
- Smoked or baked tofu is handy for picnics or travel.
- Non-GMO whole soybeans are available online and cook up quickly in your pressure cooker.
- Toasted soybeans are like dry-roasted peanuts. You can toast them yourself in the oven or purchase them online.

POWER FOODS FOR LOWERING CHOLESTEROL

At the University of Toronto, Dr. David Jenkins and his research team set about identifying the most powerful foods for cholesterol control. They started by eliminating foods that contain cholesterol and any significant amount of saturated fat. That meant eliminating meat, dairy products, and eggs. They then *added* certain foods known to have cholesterol-lowering effects. The team came up with a "portfolio" of foods that they put to the test. The list is similar to the list of weight-loss foods, with just a few differences:

- Soy protein: Soy milk and burgers, hot dogs, and deli slices made of soy.
- Soluble fiber: Oats, barley, okra, eggplant, and beans. The participants were also given psyllium fiber (a supplement marketed as Metamucil).
- Almonds: A small serving (about an ounce) of almonds per day.
- A special plant-sterol margarine (e.g., Benecol).

For example, a portfolio breakfast might include oat bran cereal topped with blueberries and served with soy milk. Lunch might include lentil soup, a soy hot dog, and a salad of lettuce, tomato, and cucumber. Dinner could be a tofu bake with ratatouille, with a side of pearled barley, broccoli, or cauliflower. Snacks could include an apple or other fruit, a glass of soy milk, or a small serving of almonds.

This portfolio diet proved to be as powerful as cholesterol-lowering drugs, reducing LDL cholesterol ("bad" cholesterol) levels by about 30 percent in four weeks. All that, with no negative effects.[27]

Grains

Cultures that tend to stay slim usually have a grain as their staple. This is particularly noticeable in Asia where rice has been a principal food for millennia. In recent decades, as the rice-based diet has given way to meatier fare, much of this advantage has been forfeited.

Grains are not just a healthy choice, they are also a culinary delight, transforming into muffins, pancakes, breakfast cereals, breads, polenta, spaghetti, risotto, cakes, and cookies. Some are, of course, healthier than others, depending on what else went into them and what was taken out. For example, whole grains have fiber; refined grains have lost much of it. With a few tricks, they can *all* be healthy. Let's look at some grains with particular health power.

The Power of Rice

As we've seen, rice has long been the staple food of the world's slimmest countries. It is a snap to make on the stovetop or in a rice cooker. Flavor it with fresh herbs, cloves, dried fruit, peas, or whatever you like, and use it as a side dish or at the center of the plate—for example, in vegetable biryani.

There are some major advantages to choosing brown rice. The tan coating is where the fiber and many nutrients are. All of that is stripped away in making white rice. Because its shelf life is shorter than that of white rice and it is slightly trickier to cook, brown rice tends to be neglected. In the recipe section, I will share a particularly good way to cook brown rice that involves briefly toasting it first. You will love it.

Whole grains, like brown rice, fill you up with relatively few calories. Then, they trap some of the calories you did take in and carry them out with the wastes so you cannot absorb them. As you will recall, brown rice was one of the foods specifically shown to trap calories in the Tufts University studies.[28] Whole grains also boost your metabolism in the after-meal hours. All this makes for easy weight loss.[29]

That said, white rice is not your enemy. It beats Velveeta and chicken wings any day, because it is rich in healthful complex carbohydrates, has practically no fat, and is naturally modest in calories. Asian populations consuming white rice at more or less every meal stayed slim—until American fast-food chains invaded, and burgers and cheese began to push rice off the plate. So if you find yourself at a restaurant that serves only white rice, don't storm out. The white rice will be far better than what other people are eating.

Despite its naturally reticent nature, rice finds its way into wonderful dishes: Red Pepper and Artichoke Paella, a Rainbow Fajita Bowl, Asian-Inspired Rice Salad with Orange Ginger Dressing, a Pinto Picnic Salad, a Garlic Cauliflower Risotto, and Sheet Pan Broccoli and Tofu Teriyaki.

Like all plants, rice picks up whatever elements are in the soil. Unfortunately, some areas of the southern United States and elsewhere have lingering arsenic residues from timber production and agriculture that can end up in rice. The concern is that arsenic is linked to cancer. Luckily, large research studies have shown no increased cancer incidence among people eating rice.[30] In any case, rice from California, India, and Pakistan tends to be cleaner. Boiling rice in excess water allows arsenic traces to pass into the cooking water, which is then discarded.

Tips for Buying and Storing Rice

- Try short-grain brown rice for a nutty texture. See the simple and quick recipe for Perfect Brown Rice.
- Red rice is similar to brown rice but gets its color from natural anthocyanins—cousins of the pigment in berries.
- Red *yeast* rice is just white rice that draws its color from being cultivated with *Monascus purpureus*, a mold that produces a cholesterol-lowering compound identical to the commercial drug lovastatin.
- Rice in the bulk section of stores is especially economical.
- Organic varieties are always best.
- Barley and millet combine well with rice in the cooking process.

The Power of Oats, Corn, and Wheat

Morning oats really do lower cholesterol. Their fiber is also an appetite-tamer, and their nutrient mix will rev up your metabolism all morning. To do oats right, start with old-fashioned or steel-cut oats, rather than instant or "minute" varieties. They will still cook up quickly and have a significant appetite-taming effect. The package instructions tell you to boil the water, then pour in the oats. That's fine, if you like your oats hard as gravel. Here is a better way: Pour the oats and water into the pan *before* you turn on the heat. That way, the oats will turn out creamy.

Be sure to *measure*. You can eyeball quantities in making spaghetti sauce or soup, but oatmeal has to be measured to avoid being soupy or stiff.

Oats are like the little girl who loves to wear a tiara. They are eager to be adorned with toppings: raisins, dates, berries, or sliced bananas, and don't forget the cinnamon.

Like all corn dishes, grits are Native American in origin. If you choose stone-ground grits, as opposed to the quicker-cooking varieties, you'll take advantage of the entire kernel, natural fiber and all.

Like oats, grits love toppings. Skip the butter, of course, but there is no shortage of healthful additions. Make them sweet with raisins, berries, brown sugar, cinnamon, maple syrup, or jam. Or make them savory with herbs, tomatoes, roasted red peppers, caramelized onion, or scallions. Many people like them with just black pepper.

The wheat-based equivalent is Cream of Wheat, which can be garnished in the same way and has many of the same health benefits.

Success!

Janelle was forty-eight years old when she decided it was time to take better care of herself. Her children were grown, and she was comfortable in her job. But when she looked in the mirror, she did not see the woman she wanted to be. She decided to get some advice.

There was a gym next door to her office, and the membership was free for the first month. She joined and got some coaching from a friendly man about half her age. He gave her a list of exercises to try and, if weight loss was her goal, he encouraged her to keep her diet "lean." That meant chicken, fish, egg whites, and avoiding carbs. He counseled her to avoid bread and pasta and to be careful about fruit. "And don't eat anything white: no flour, potatoes, sugar, or salt," he said.

She was not entirely sure about this. After all, her coach did not look especially healthy. Nonetheless, she had read similar advice in magazines and decided it was worth a try. She cleaned out her shelves and gave away her pasta, rice, bread, and breakfast cereals. It seemed peculiar to give away an unopened box of healthy-looking oatmeal, but she resolved to do her best.

After two months, she could not take it anymore. Her weight loss was minimal and the diet seemed far too restrictive.

It was around that time that she heard about our research study, in which we were testing what was essentially the opposite of what she had been doing. It not only allowed but *encouraged* participants to bring foods into their lives. Grains, beans, pasta, breads, and potatoes were on the good list, as were a great many other foods she liked.

She joined the study and quickly switched gears. She abandoned the notion of avoiding carbs and ate an abundance of healthful foods, following the approach described in this book. Within the first week, the weight started to come off, and it continued week by week. More important, she *felt* good. Her spark was coming back. She continued to exercise at the gym, but did not follow the gym's diet advice. Her gym instructor watched her progress over time and smiled, imagining that his guidance had worked for her. Only much later did she tell him what she had done. At first, he found it impossible to believe that grains and carbs in general could fit into a healthy diet. But she referred him to a class we sponsored for health professionals, which he attended. He also saw a film called *The Game Changers*, about athletes following plant-based diets. He ended up trying it and was surprised to see that he felt better, too. It energized his work. Janelle probably could have charged him for her advice. But she was just happy for his success, and hers.

The Power of Pasta

Picture an Italian restaurant. Your server lights a candle and pours you a glass of Chianti. Next comes a pretty plate of bruschetta, followed by a a cup of Tuscan lentil soup or pasta e fagioli and a salad of butter lettuce and radicchio topped with grape tomatoes.

Then the chef brings his signature pasta arrabbiata. *Arrabbiata* is the Italian word for "angry," as in "spicy," although only mildly so. Let's just say your pasta is feeling assertive. Your server follows up with garlic spinach and chard. At dinner's end, you'll have an espresso.

If you had the idea that this was a fattening meal or that pasta in general is loaded with calories, well, *permettimi di correggerti*! Typical spaghetti, macaroni, penne, or angel hair noodles are just ground-up wheat. Their healthy mix of complex carbohydrate and protein (about 15 percent) is exactly the combination for a good after-meal burn. Whole-wheat pasta has more fiber than white pasta, of course, which is an advantage. But whether it's white or whole-grain, the fattening part of a typical pasta dish is the *toppings*—meat, cheese, and oil. With healthier toppings, you're fine.

Let's see if that's true. Hop in the car, and let's go to Olive Garden, the Italian-inspired chain restaurant. Let's say you were to choose spaghetti with meat sauce. After the server takes your order, we log on to the US Department of Agriculture Food Data Central database, which tells us that Olive Garden Spaghetti with Meat Sauce has 121 calories in every 100-gram ladleful. Okay, wait. The server has not yet put in our order, so let's check Spaghetti with Pomodoro Sauce (that is, tomato sauce). It's basically the same thing, but the fat is cut nearly in half and the calories are down to 102. Waiter, can I change my order? Over the course of a day or a week, little differences like this add up. A 2018 meta-analysis showed that, as part of an otherwise healthy diet, pasta is consistently associated with weight loss.[31] That bears repeating: Pasta equals weight loss.

Our chef's arrabbiata sauce is made from diced tomatoes, tomato paste, basil, lemon juice, Italian seasoning, onion, and garlic, plus however many red pepper flakes he was in the mood to stir in, plus a splash of wine, a spoon of sugar, and parsley for a garnish.

Creative chefs also stuff ravioli or pasta shells with spinach, kale, crumbled tofu, mushrooms, pumpkin, butternut squash, and season with garlic, basil, sage, thyme, nutritional yeast, and other ingredients, and you can, too. There are endless possibilities.

There are, of course, countless other grains, from amaranth to quinoa, and it's great to experiment with them and see which ones you like best.

WHAT ABOUT GLUTEN?

Gluten is a natural protein that bakers love. It stretches. That means it makes perfect pizza dough, pie crust, and soft bread. Gluten is found in wheat, barley, rye, triticale, malted grains, and brewer's yeast (which contains gluten from barley), and is the protein in seitan, a common meat substitute.

However, just as some people are allergic to peanuts or strawberries, about 1 percent of the population has an auto-immune reaction to gluten, called *celiac disease*, manifesting as severe and even life-threatening intestinal symptoms. People with celiac disease must avoid gluten. In addition, some people, perhaps one in ten, find that avoiding gluten gives them better digestion or makes them feel better in other ways. For everyone else, avoiding gluten has no apparent benefit. If that includes you, get to know bread and pasta again. These centuries-old healthful foods have missed you. Nonetheless, the inexplicably large market for gluten-free products has caused manufacturers to come up with rice-based pizza crusts and all manner of other new products that are interesting to try.

Yippee! A Bowl of Cereal!

Some people have come to fear grains, imagining that their natural carbohydrates might be fattening. The truth is just the opposite. Whole grains are modest in calories and bring you plenty of calorie-trapping fiber.

I was recently speaking with a couple who were interested in losing weight. In discussing breakfast options, they were floored—and delighted—that my recommendations would allow a bowl of cereal.

"Sure, cereal is fine," I said.

"Really? You mean, like cornflakes? Wheaties? Cheerios?" They looked like they had just won the lottery.

"No problem. Cereal's okay. Knock yourself out." I was puzzled as to why this was such a cause for celebration.

She explained: "We have been doing low-carb basically forever. No bread, no fruit, no pasta, no cookies, no this, no that. A bowl of cereal is something I never thought I would ever have again. I really can't believe it."

I realized that some fad diets turn reality on its head, punishing people for wanting simple, healthful foods. Yes, we should consider *what goes on* the cereal, but cereal itself is A-OK.

Vegetables

In the heart of Paris, chef Alain Passard revolutionized the culinary world. In 1986, he purchased a restaurant across the street from the Musée Rodin and renamed it Arpège, meaning "arpeggio." It soon won its first Michelin star, then its second, and then its third. It is one of only ten restaurants in Paris that hold this distinction.

Passard soon found cooking meat to be dull and uninspiring and began to be taken with the artistry of vegetables. While many American restaurants view vegetables as something to be dumped out of a number ten tin can, French chefs view them differently. They buy them at local markets, carefully evaluating their freshness and choosing only the best.

"The best cookbook ever written," Passard said, "was by Mother Nature herself." He created his own gardens to grow carrots, cabbages, asparagus, leeks, celeriac, and aromatic herbs. Vegetables became the focus of Arpège's menu: visually beautiful, with delicate tastes, and submitting readily to seasonings and cooking techniques. In turn, other leading chefs took a similar path, away from meat and toward plants.

For health and weight loss, vegetables are powerful. They have calorie-trapping fiber, a surprisingly large amount of protein, ounce for ounce, and almost no fat. Once liberated from the usual oil, fatback, or cheese sauce that many people have grown up with, vegetables come into their own. In the bargain, they boost heart health, cut cancer risk, and bring myriad other benefits.

Let's examine some stars in the vegetable world and see how to give them the respect they deserve.

The Power of Green Vegetables

Cruciferous vegetables deserve special attention. Named for their cross-shaped flowers, this group includes broccoli, kale, collards, cabbage, cauliflower, and brussels sprouts, among others. While many people choose them for their highly absorbable calcium, they also have healthful iron, fiber, traces of healthy omega-3 fats, and a special natural compound called *sulforaphane* that enhances your body's detoxing ability by boosting the liver enzymes that neutralize toxic compounds.

As you will recall from chapter 2, the Harvard research team put cruciferous vegetables high on the weight-loss list; that is, the more people added them to their meals, the more weight they lost. Include them generously in your routine. Their high-fiber content, combined with their very low fat content, makes them very effective.

Some people find green vegetables to be a bit bitter. If this includes you, try these simple tips:

- Cook them thoroughly to soften their taste and improve digestibility.
- Top them with Bragg Liquid Aminos, which is waiting for you next to the soy sauce at health food stores.
- Spritz them with lemon juice. For some reason, the sourness of lemon juice combines with the faintly bitter taste of vegetables and turns everything sweet and delectable. You can do the same with a flavorful vinegar—seasoned rice vinegar, malt vinegar, or any other.
- By the way, before slicing your lemon, roll it on the countertop to break up the fibers. Then, cut it *lengthwise*, which makes it easier to squeeze.

Apart from cruciferous vegetables, enjoy the full range of other green delights: Chinese vegetables, like bok choy, Morning Glory (choy sum), and Chinese spinach (available with many more wonderful greens in your local Asian market); as well as watercress, asparagus, spinach, dandelion leaves, Swiss chard, lettuce of all varieties, and everything else the produce department has to offer.

The Family That Never Ate Vegetables

One of our research participants, a man in his early forties, told me, "We don't eat vegetables—we just don't." He was referring to himself and his teenage children, whom he was raising as a single parent. He had nothing against vegetables. They were just not part of their routine.

His family was not alone. An average American might get a serving or two a day, if we count potato chips. But for many people, the vegetable aisle is not a shopping destination. Given vegetables' health value, though, I suggested he explore a few choices and see what he might find. As he left our offices, it seemed he was not in the least bit intrigued by my suggestion.

As it turned out, I had misjudged him. He went home, reread the materials we had provided about vegetables, health, and weight loss—everything you already know—and he decided to experiment. He picked up some frozen broccoli florets, which were easy to cook, and topped them with rice vinegar, as I had suggested. He bought some Swiss chard, steamed it, and then added Bragg Liquid Aminos. His fifteen-year-old son was not keen on either of these, but quite liked vegetables that were not cooked—salad greens of all kinds, carrots, and celery—so Dad kept them on hand. His eighteen-year-old daughter liked anything she could put in a smoothie: spinach, kale, or chard, along with fruits and soy milk.

As time went on, he had great success—not just with vegetables, but with a range of simple, healthy foods he had not explored previously. He revamped his diet and lost about sixty-five pounds over several months. Later on, I asked what had made him turn the corner and decide to try out these new foods.

"Let me show you," he said. He reached into his pocket and pulled out his wallet. In it was a crumpled picture of his wife, who had died some years ago, and their two children. "If it was just me, Doc, I wouldn't really care. But I need to be there for them, and I want them healthy, too. And as you go on, you like it. The food is good."

The Power of Orange Vegetables

Earlier, we were bragging about mangoes, papayas, and the beta-carotene they hold. You'll recall that a Florida research team found that beta-carotene promotes fat loss, especially for abdominal fat. It will not surprise you that there is even more beta-carotene in sweet potatoes and carrots. And both are naturally low in calories—about 115 calories in an entire sweet potato and only 70 calories in a cup of chopped carrots. If we can resist the urge to slather butter all over the top, these are great foods.

In the produce aisle, sweet potatoes are a simple, basic food. In the kitchen, a chef will use them the way an artist uses oil paints. Here are some chef d'oeuvres you can create at home.

For breakfast, sweet potato muffins made with nutmeg, cinnamon, and raisins are delicious. Or how about sweet potato hash with red and green peppers, garlic, and onions? Or a breakfast pudding of blended sweet potato, rolled oats, cinnamon, maple syrup, and a bit of vanilla soy milk?

For a fun treat, make sweet potato toasts: Just pop some sprouted-grain bread in the toaster, then top it with a mash of sweet potatoes, lemon juice, salt, and pepper, and sprinkle on a couple of sliced black olives.

At lunch, a sweet potato burrito is quick and delicious. Just stuff a whole-wheat tortilla with mashed sweet potato, corn, black beans, and green onions, and flavor with lime juice and chili powder. Sprinkle on shredded lettuce and salsa, and you've got it.

Sweet potato can also be mixed into hummus and used as a dip or sandwich filling. If you have not yet tried making your own hummus, it's quick, fun, healthy, and almost free.

Needless to say, you can make sweet potato fries. Bake them, don't fry them, and sprinkle them with parsley, thyme, cracked pepper, smoked paprika, cumin, garlic, and cayenne.

At dinner, we can get a little fancy with a shepherd's pie, starting with mushrooms, peas or lentils, and spices, and layered with a crisp sweet potato topping. We can create an easy sweet potato casserole with a bit of maple syrup, cinnamon, ginger, apricots, orange zest, and a sprinkle of pumpkin seeds on top, and pop it in the oven to turn golden brown.

We might also want to just keep it simple. Starting with a baked sweet potato, top it with black beans, salsa, corn, cilantro, chopped tomatoes, and scallions, or mash it with salt and pepper, and sprinkle with toasted sage leaves. Or eat this sweet treat just as it comes.

ORANGE + GREEN

A healthy dinner trick is to pair an orange vegetable with a green vegetable: sweet potato with broccoli, or steamed carrots with Swiss chard, topped with a spray of Bragg Liquid Aminos.

The slight sweetness of the orange vegetable that comes out during the cooking process acts like a seasoning for the green vegetable. Nutritionally, they complement each other, creating a powerhouse for health.

Not to be outdone, carrots are versatile, too. They can start your day as carrot juice, with apple, ginger, or whatever other additions you might like.

Carrot ginger soup is delicious, so easy to make, and very pretty, sprinkled with scallions.

You can use carrots as snacks, of course. A fun lunch for kids and adults is a carrot chili dog. You just boil carrots until soft, then marinate them in soy sauce, garlic, black pepper, and liquid smoke, grill them, and serve in a hot dog bun with your favorite toppings: ketchup, mustard, relish, tomatoes, onions, hot peppers, and, if you like, baked beans.

Carrot cake is delicious flavored with ginger, nutmeg, and a touch of cinnamon and brown sugar. It is an easy matter to replace the oil or butter with unsweetened applesauce, mashed banana, silken tofu, or pumpkin puree, and to replace the eggs with unsweetened applesauce, mashed banana, or chia seeds.

The point, of course, is to use foods that have the appetite-taming, calorie-trapping, and metabolism-boosting effects—and sweet potatoes and carrots have all three. The recipes in this book are so delicious, you will want to put them to work again and again.

ORANGE IS THE NEW BLUE

You may have heard of the Blue Zones—places where people have extraordinary longevity. The concept was born as researcher, athlete, and author Dan Buettner and his *National*

Geographic team tracked longevity on a world map, marking in blue those locations where people lived longest.

The place with more centenarians per capita than any other turned out to be Okinawa, at the southern end of Japan. The region's dietary staple is not rice, fish, or whatever other Japanese traditions might come to mind. It is the sweet potato. This humble food that Americans think about at Thanksgiving and ignore the rest of the year is front and center in the traditional Okinawan diet.[32] It provides more than half their calories. The common variety there is more purple than orange, but you can pick up sweet potatoes at your local grocery and enjoy their health benefits any time of year.

Butternut Squash

Is it a vegetable or a fruit? And is that really beta-carotene?

Botanically, a squash is a fruit, but because it is not as sweet as an orange or apple, people use it in dishes as if it were a starchy vegetable. And yes, that's beta-carotene, and lots of it.

Let's augment squash's beta-carotene and appetite-taming fiber by roasting it and adding cinnamon (of course), plus fresh rosemary, and maple syrup, agave, or molasses. It will be irresistible.

Butternut squash soup is a real gift. You will find convenient canned versions, with or without added salt. And it's a snap to make your own: Just cut the squash into cubes (or buy it pre-cut), roast in the oven with chunks of onion and apple, then pop it in a blender with vegetable broth, and whatever spices call to you—perhaps curry powder, thyme, or nutmeg, and you've got soup. Keep it in your refrigerator and, when you're hungry, just heat and enjoy. You might top it with parsley, cilantro, or pumpkin seeds.

A butternut squash may be an awkward shape, but cutting it is actually very easy. Here's how:

1. Cut off both ends, then, with a vegetable peeler, shave off the skin.
2. With a crosswise slice, cut the elongated neck off the round body.
3. Stand the neck on one end and cut it in half, and do the same to the body, then scoop out the seeds.
4. Place each piece on a cutting board, cut side down, and slice it crosswise, then lengthwise, making cubes.

Sweet Potatoes, Black Beans, and Love

Stefanie Ignoffo grew up in a small town in northern Illinois, not far from the Wisconsin border. Weight issues started early. "By the time I was in the third grade, I was the 'chunky kid,'" she said. According to her pediatrician, her weight problem was hereditary. As she grew up, things did not get better. At twenty-one, she carried 200 pounds on her five-foot-two-inch frame. Her blood pressure climbed, and that, apparently, was hereditary, too.

She dieted repeatedly, losing weight that inevitably came back. For her wedding at age twenty-three, she managed to trim down to 173 pounds, but the weight crept back on, and when she became pregnant, she gained considerably more. Eventually, she reached 280 pounds.

Her husband had weight issues, too. Together they attended Weight Watchers and ate low-fat cottage cheese, lean chicken, ground turkey, eggs, and fruits and vegetables. But the foods were not filling, and their diets did not work well in social situations. They avoided restaurants. They became convinced that *they* were the problem: Their willpower was just inadequate.

In 2012, their fifteen-year-old daughter decided to stop eating animal products for ethical reasons. Her initial diet explorations were awkward, relying on convenience foods, but she gradually began to cook and find healthier options.

Some months later, Stefanie decided to do the same. Out with the meat, dairy products, eggs, and greasy foods. And this opened the door to an exploration of the power of vegetables, fruits, whole grains, and beans.

In the kitchen, they made stir-fries, lasagna, and grain bowls with beans and vegetables. They combined the power of sweet potatoes, black beans, and oats in a sweet potato and black bean burger seasoned with garlic and onion powder. They began to make their own sushi with cucumbers, julienned carrots, jicama, tomatoes, and tofu marinated with seaweed.

Within days, Stefanie's weight started coming off. Within two weeks, her blood pressure had improved to the point where she was able to discontinue her medications.

The whole family joined in the experiment: Stefanie, her husband, and their children, who were ages thirteen, fifteen, and seventeen. They had more energy and were sleeping better. The children's acne cleared up.

Their pediatrician was against the diet, saying they would not get enough protein, which left Stefanie feeling intimidated but undaunted. They kept at it. Stefanie took on the role of an encouraging coach. Rather than timidly suggesting foods that her children might try, she really encouraged them. "We are taught to buckle our kids up in the car and put a helmet on them when they ride their bikes," she said. "We can't let ourselves get overly permissive with things that can hurt them, whether it's cigarettes, drugs, or unhealthy foods."

In ten months, the family had lost 250 pounds. Stefanie got down to 132 pounds and felt wonderful. As they became healthier, they found they had the energy to become more physically active, and they love biking together.

Stefanie began to help other people to lose weight and improve their health. Eventually, she decided to start a non-profit called Plantspiration and became a Food for Life instructor with the Physicians Committee. "I got a second chance at life," she says. "I want to tell as many people as I can."

The Power of Potatoes

With only about 150 calories or so and virtually no fat, potatoes' appetite-taming and metabolism-boosting abilities have helped many people lose weight. Perhaps the most famous was magician Penn Jillette, who, motivated by a heart condition, used an all-potato diet to jump-start his weight loss. He gradually added in other vegetables, fruits, and grains, while avoiding animal products, added oils, and refined grains, and eventually lost more than one hundred pounds.

Andrew Taylor, of Melbourne, Australia, followed suit. At 334 pounds, he felt he needed to tackle food addiction, and decided to limit himself to potatoes and sweet potatoes, usually baked or boiled, with added spices, herbs, and fat-free sauces, or mashed with added soy milk, plus a vitamin B_{12} supplement. He went through eight or nine pounds of potatoes per day.

Along the way, he surprised his doctor with his robust health. His cholesterol levels improved, his mood and sleep improved, his strength and energy got better, and he lost 114 pounds.

I am not recommending that you do the same, although you could if you wanted to. The point is this: Potatoes are healthful choices. The problem is what we add to them. Cooking oil, butter, gravy, sour cream, and cheese or cheese sauce pack a lot of calories, and unfortunately that is how most people eat them. Harvard researchers found that the way Americans tend to eat potatoes can spell weight *gain*.[33] Instead, let the potato's natural healthfulness shine through. Here are some examples.

Hash browns and home fries can be browned to perfection without oil and topped with onions, chives, green peppers, jalapeños, tomatoes, or endless other additions.

Potato salad is a perfect summer treat, with celery, parsley, green onions, rice vinegar, chopped dill pickles, chives, and Dijon mustard. If you like, add the flavors of green and red peppers, olives, white beans, garlic, lime juice, salt, pepper, and a touch of oil-free vegan mayo.

Roasted potatoes with rosemary, thyme, garlic, salt, and pepper emerge from the oven bursting with flavor.

Baked potatoes can be topped with grilled mushrooms, mustard, soy sauce, salsa, broccoli, baked beans, or veggie chili. If you like, scoop out the inside, mash with chives and pepper, and return it to the jacket.

Mashed Yukon golds are great with mushroom gravy, garlic salt, pepper, or miso.

On the Champs-Élysées, they are *pommes vapeur*. In London, they are steamed new potatoes. Whatever you call them, top these little white potatoes with mint sauce: a dressing made of vinegar, chopped fresh mint, and a pinch of sugar.

French fries are still on the menu. They are baked, not fried, and you will soon come to prefer the non-oil version. If you have an air fryer, French fries are a snap.

Potatoes lend themselves to other delights: They can top a shepherd's pie (a little nutritional yeast or a brushing of plant-based milk will deliver a delightful brown crust to them). They will jump into a vegetable stew, stuff a tortilla along with caramelized onions, or join spinach and tomatoes to create a savory Indian curry.

Authentic Mashed Potatoes

There's nothing wrong with instant mashed potatoes. However, it is easy to make mashed potatoes from scratch, and you will taste the difference. Start with Yukon golds, russets, or both together. Just peel, cube, and boil them, then mash. Alternatively, you might try roasting them in their skins, then removing the skins and mashing them.

Either way, keep it low-tech and use a potato masher. If there is a lump or two left, that just proves they really are homemade. Do not use a food processor or immersion blender; the potatoes will come out gluey. This can even happen if you mash them too hard by hand, so don't mash potatoes if you have just been in an argument.

Tips for Buying and Storing Potatoes

- Use the best potato for the job. There are seven categories based on color and shape: "Russet" is an old word for reddish-brown. There are also red, white, yellow, and blue/purple potatoes, plus fingerling and petite potatoes.
  - For baking, russets are your best friend, but red and Yukon gold work great, too. Choose potatoes that are all medium-sized; they will bake well and be ready to come out of the oven at the same time.
  - For boiling, you might like new potatoes. They are harvested before full maturity, so their peels are more delicate. New potatoes are also great for steaming, ready to be sprinkled with vinegar, mint, parsley, or chives.
  - For mashed potatoes, Yukon golds are great, and russets are, too.
  - For roasting, use yellow potatoes.
- Favor organic varieties. Conventionally grown potatoes are often chemically treated.

- Don't buy potatoes with cuts, blemishes, green patches, or significant sprouting. What you see on the outside is a hint at what's inside.

- Do not wash potatoes before storage; dampness is your enemy. Wash them just before you use them, even if you plan to peel them.

- For the same reason, let potatoes breathe. Keep them in an open bowl or open paper bag so that moisture does not accumulate.

- Potatoes kept at room temperature should be used within a couple of weeks, before they get ideas about sprouting or shriveling. If you are keeping them longer, they do best at cool temperatures, around 45 to 50 degrees Fahrenheit, but do not put them in the refrigerator. That's too cold.

The Power of Sea Vegetables

Many people are not yet familiar with the wondrous vegetables that grow below sea level. That's a shame, because sea vegetables have something that is rare in the culinary world. Your thyroid gland needs iodine to make thyroid hormone, and thyroid hormone is key to powering up your metabolism. Optimally, you need 150 micrograms of iodine per day, and sea vegetables go a long way toward getting you there. Let me recommend three that you will want to get to know:

Nori is the wrap you typically see on a sushi roll. At a sushi bar, skip the fish sushi and have a cucumber roll, asparagus roll, or sweet potato roll. Suddenly, you have combined the appetite-taming fiber of vegetables with nori's metabolism-boosting iodine and the shaved ginger topping, which has weight-loss properties of its own.

Nori also makes a clever seasoning. In a mock tuna salad, mashed chickpeas substitute for tuna, and a sprinkle of crumbled nori brings in the flavor of the sea. You can do the same to simulate crab cakes or clam chowder. Nori is also sold in sheets as a salty snack.

You will also want to get to know **wakame** (pronounced "walk a may"), which is commonly used in miso soup and seaweed salad; and **arame** (pronounced "air a may"), a very light sea vegetable that beautifully enhances a cucumber salad, as you will see in the recipe section.

Combining the Power Foods

Now that you know about the individual foods and ingredients that will help you lose weight, let's combine their effects for real power: A blueberry muffin combines the power of anthocyanins, fiber, and complex carbohydrate. A cup of baked beans combines fiber and ginger. A vegetable stir-fry combines the power of brown rice, cruciferous vegetables, spices, and many other ingredients. The recipe section will give you many ideas.

In the next chapter, we will see where many people go wrong. We will look at the foods that can block our weight-loss efforts and what to do about them. Then, we will plan our meals and get ready to begin!

CHAPTER 3

Foods That Are Less Healthful Than You'd Think

Red curry soup made with organic coconut oil. Wild-caught Chinook salmon. Goat cheese from the Loire Valley. Exotic, delicious, and healthy, right? Well, actually no. They will stop your weight loss in its tracks.

Of course, you knew that bacon, sausage, and pizza dripping with cheese are not slimming foods, and neither is a bucket of chicken wings. But some foods, like coconut oil, salmon, and goat cheese, are *marketed* as healthful choices. They are trendy and even "natural" sounding. But their calories pass easily into body fat, and if you are not lucky, they just park there, leaving you frustrated. Along the way, they can damage your health.

There are similar problems with many everyday foods: cheddar cheese, peanut butter, or a breakfast of avocado toast. This chapter shows why these foods counteract your weight-loss efforts and what to choose instead.

Let's look at several common foods that are less healthy than you might think.

Animal Protein

Some people imagine that protein causes weight loss. They load up on egg whites and chicken breast and hope for the best. It does not work very well. What is worse, new research has shown a surprising side of animal protein.

Schoolchildren are taught that animal protein is *complete* protein and superior to whatever protein might come from plants. Athletes are given the same message. Meat, dairy, and eggs give you "better quality" protein, compared with the "incomplete" proteins in beans or whole grains—at least that was the common idea until very recently. It has turned out to be entirely mistaken. Not only can you get all the protein you need from plant sources—we have actually known that for many years—but it turns out that animal proteins can shorten your life.

If you could look at a protein molecule under a powerful microscope, it would look like a string of beads. Each "bead" is an *amino acid*—a protein building block. In your digestive tract, the "string of beads" comes apart. The individual amino acid "beads" then pass into your bloodstream, and your body uses them to repair your body tissues and make hormones and enzymes.

Your body can actually make some of these amino acids on its own. But others, called *essential amino acids*, have to come from food. And that is what made meat, dairy products, and eggs seem superior. The proteins in animal products are rich in essential amino acids. Plants have them, too, but plants vary. Beans, for example, are higher in certain amino acids and a bit lower in others. Same for grains; they are higher in some and a bit lower in others, which led people to believe that plants could leave you missing some amino acids. Scientists assumed that, because animal products were dense in essential amino acids, they were a better choice.

Later on, it became clear that although plants vary, all plants have all the essential amino acids, and a diet based on a variety of plant foods easily provides the amino acids you need. In other words, plants have plenty of good, healthy, complete protein. You don't need animal protein at all.

In 2016, Harvard researchers went further and asked the obvious question: If animal protein is somehow superior with its high content of essential amino acids, does that translate into some measurable health advantage? To answer that question, they followed 131,342 participants from the Nurses' Health Study and Health Professionals Follow-Up Study, watching what they ate and tracking their health. What they found turned the nutrition world on its head.

It turned out that the more animal protein the research participants ate, the more likely they were to die of heart disease or stroke. That was the case for fish, poultry, eggs, and dairy products, as well as red meat. Plant proteins, on the other hand, reduced the risk of dying. To the extent people replaced animal protein with plant protein, they were less likely to die.[1] In other words, animal protein is not superior to plant protein at all. Just the opposite. It presents real health drawbacks. The next question was this: Why would animal protein be linked to premature death?

Part of the problem with animal protein is that it is usually accompanied by a fair amount of fat. A steak or burger is permeated with it. A chicken breast is, too, surprisingly enough. You might not see it but, even without the skin, about a quarter of the calories in a chicken breast come from fat.

Animal products are especially high in *saturated* fat—the "bad" fat that raises cholesterol levels and is linked to Alzheimer's disease. In contrast, plants have no cholesterol and almost no saturated fat. Instead, plant proteins combine with fiber, healthy complex carbohydrates, and vitamin C. But the Harvard researchers took all those variables into account and still found that animal protein was a problem. There was something about animal protein itself.

That led scientists to look more closely at the essential amino acids, those supposedly healthful "beads" that make up the protein chain. One is called lysine, and it is indeed more abundant in meat. However, it turns out that we need only small amounts of it. Scientists suspect that meat provides *too much* lysine, leading to heart problems, especially in people with diabetes. Other amino acids, including methionine and histidine, may be harmful in excess, and animal products have a boatload of them.

Plants contain these amino acids, too, but in quantities more appropriate to our needs. They give you the protein your body requires without overdoing it and causing harm. Take that egg-white omelet and swap it for scrambled tofu, and your odds of living longer increase. Same for fish, poultry, red meat, and dairy products. Replacing them with plant protein was associated with less risk of dying at any given time.

In truth, this was not entirely a surprise, because we had been through the same issue with iron. In the 1950s, scientists thought that the load of iron in meat or liver was an advantage. They do indeed have a lot of it, including a special form called *heme* iron, which was particularly absorbable. As time went on, however, scientists discovered that it was easy to store up too much iron, and that excess iron could cause heart disease, Alzheimer's disease, and premature aging. Plants have iron, too, but in a form that is easier for the body to regulate: We can absorb more if we need more and can reduce absorption when we already have plenty on board.

Here's the point: You already knew that animal products have cholesterol and "bad fat." But it turns out that the protein itself seems to be a problem. It may be too dense in certain essential amino acids. You will get a healthier mix of essential amino acids from a menu drawn from beans, grains, vegetables, and fruit. In 2020, researchers conducted a meta-analysis, combining the results of thirty-one cohort studies, confirming that plant proteins were better for health.[2] Other researchers agree.[3]

Animal products in general are rapidly falling out of favor for many reasons. In case we skipped over it too quickly, the fat in meat

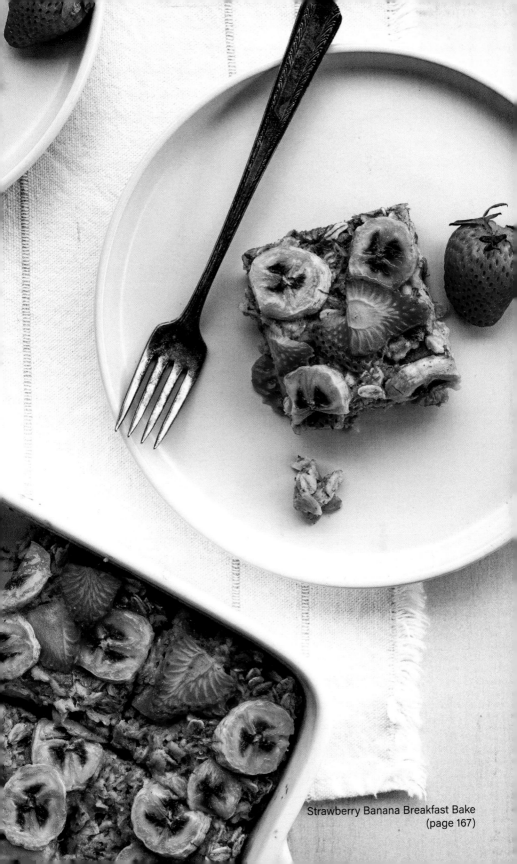

Strawberry Banana Breakfast Bake
(page 167)

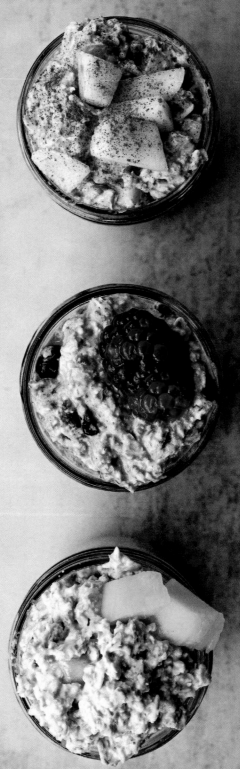

Everyday Overnight Oats Three Ways (page 168)

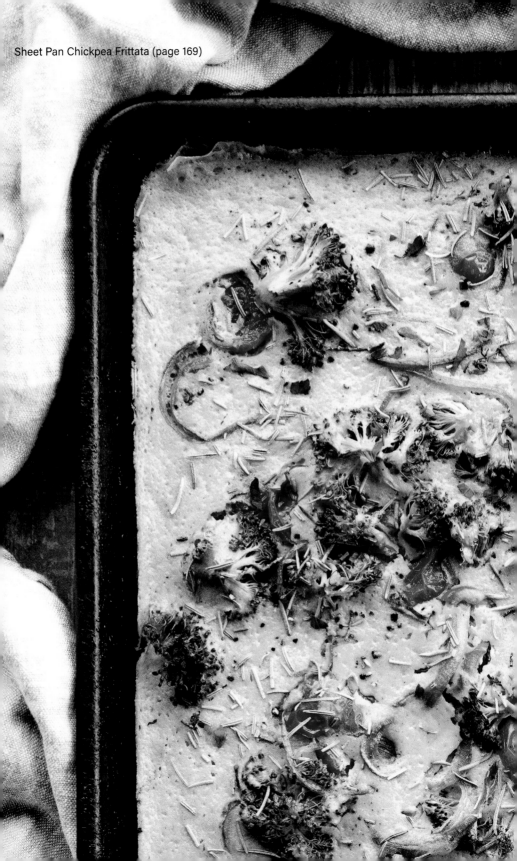

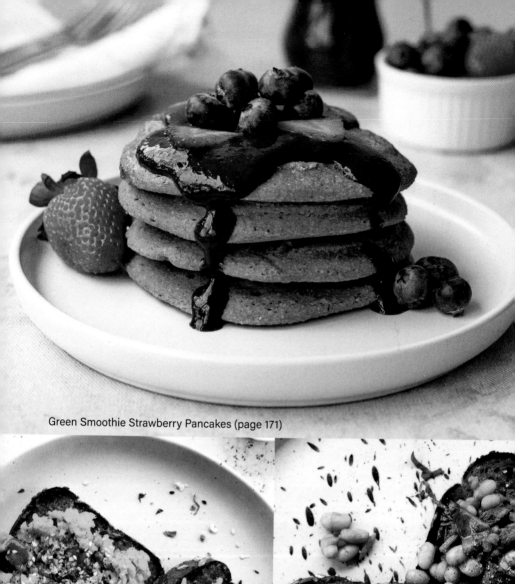

Green Smoothie Strawberry Pancakes (page 171)

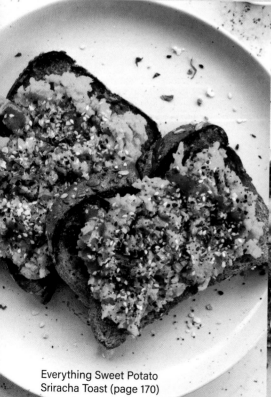

Everything Sweet Potato
Sriracha Toast (page 170)

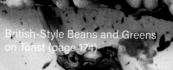

British-Style Beans and Greens
on Toast (page 174)

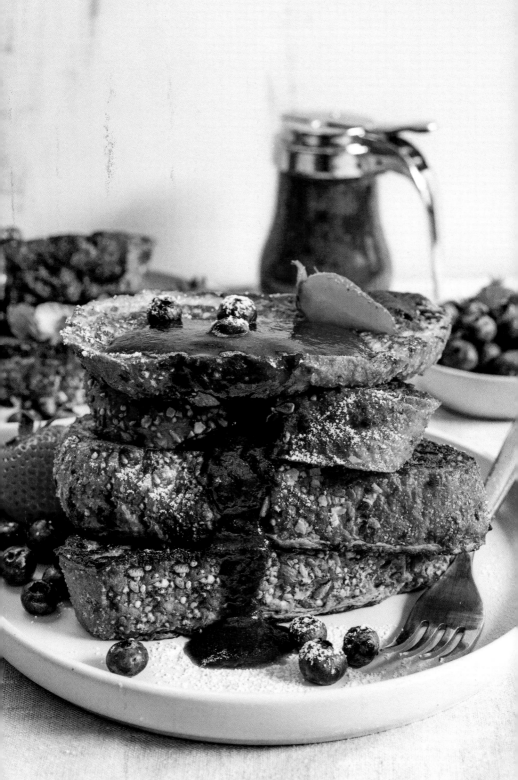

French Toast (page 182)

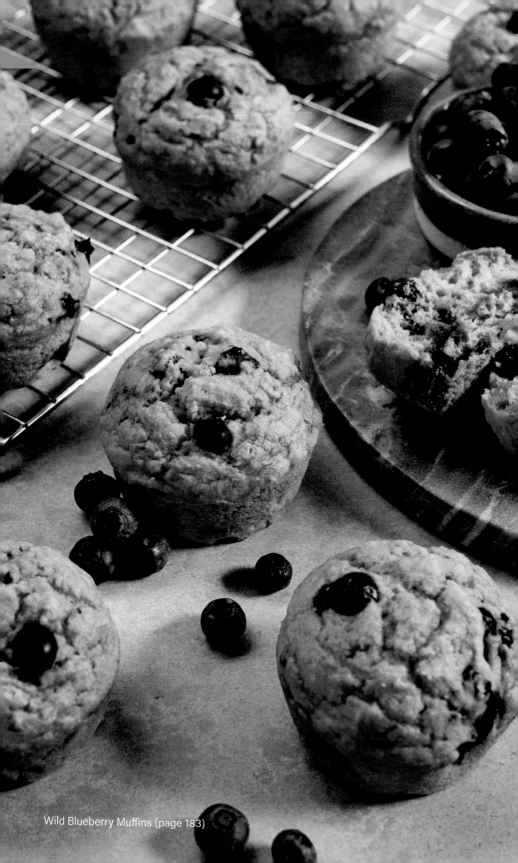

Wild Blueberry Muffins (page 183)

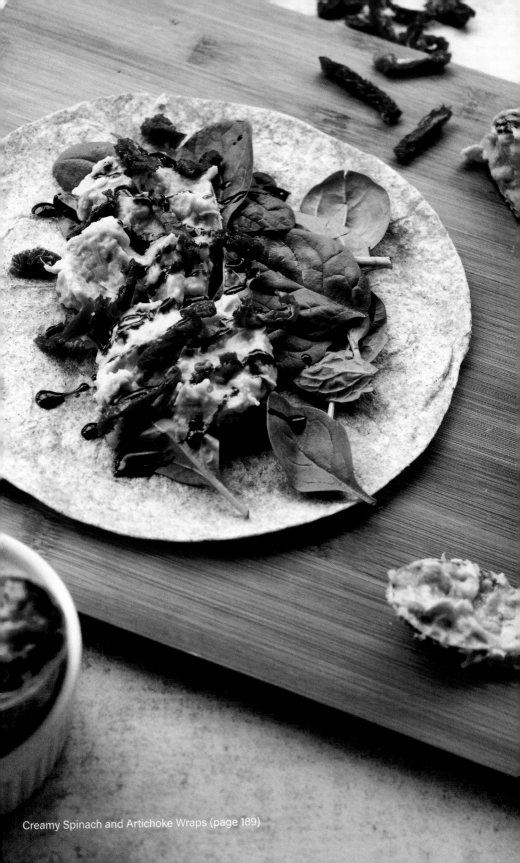

Creamy Spinach and Artichoke Wraps (page 189)

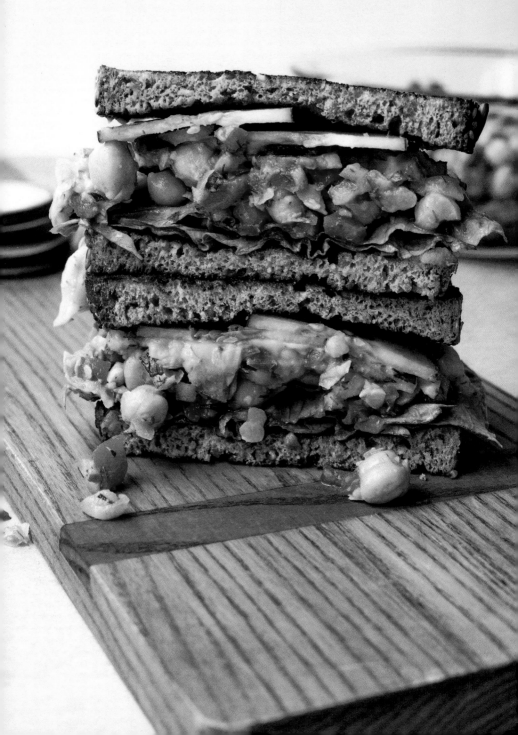

Mediterranean Chickpea Salad Sandwiches (page 190)

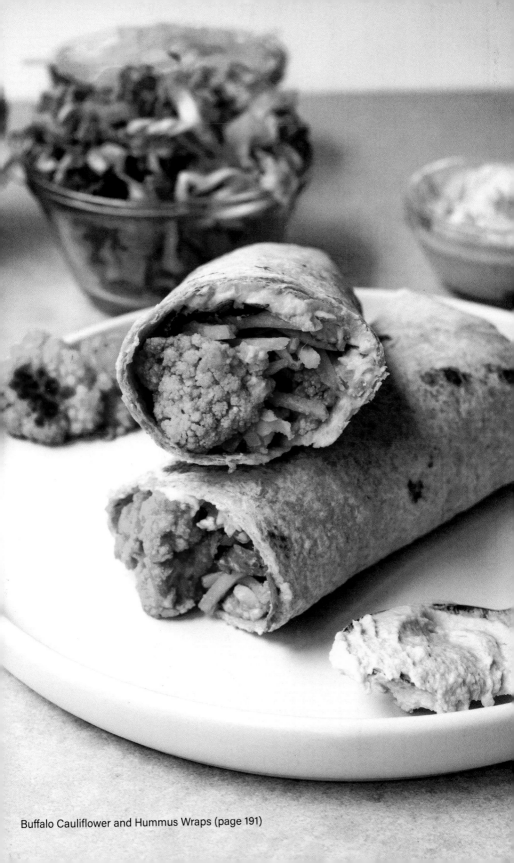

Buffalo Cauliflower and Hummus Wraps (page 191)

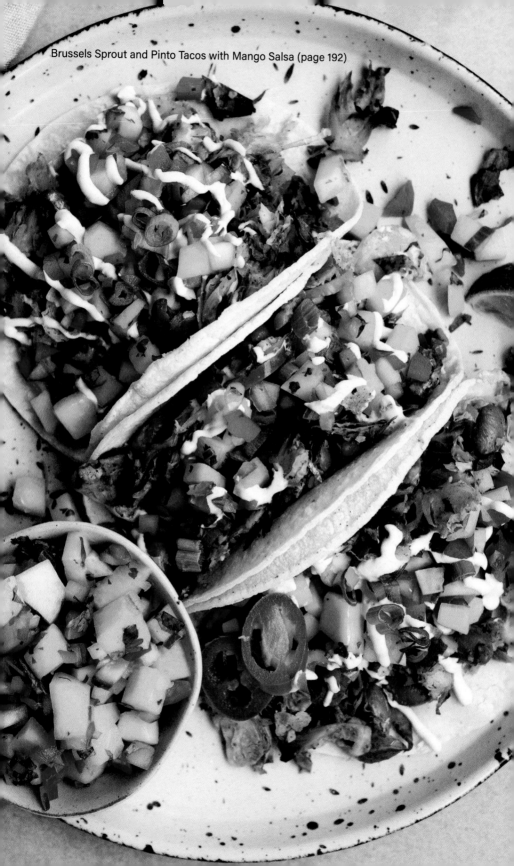

Brussels Sprout and Pinto Tacos with Mango Salsa (page 192)

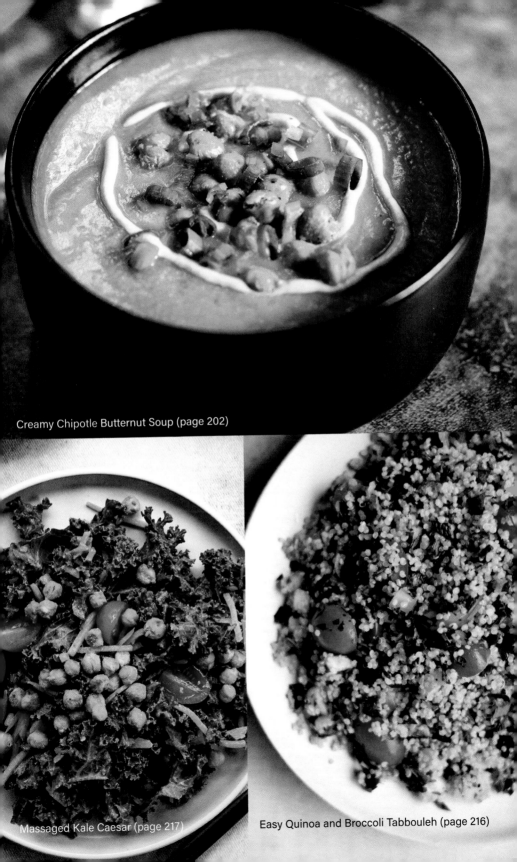

Creamy Chipotle Butternut Soup (page 202)

Massaged Kale Caesar (page 217)

Easy Quinoa and Broccoli Tabbouleh (page 216)

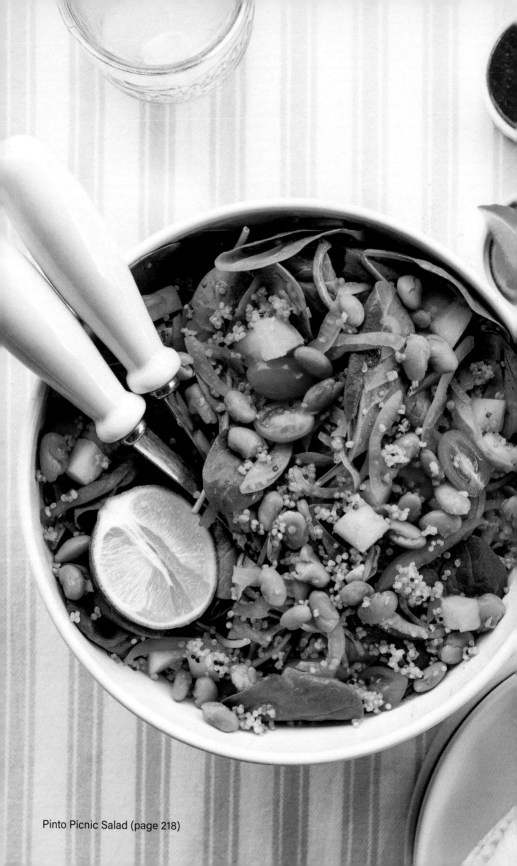

Pinto Picnic Salad (page 218)

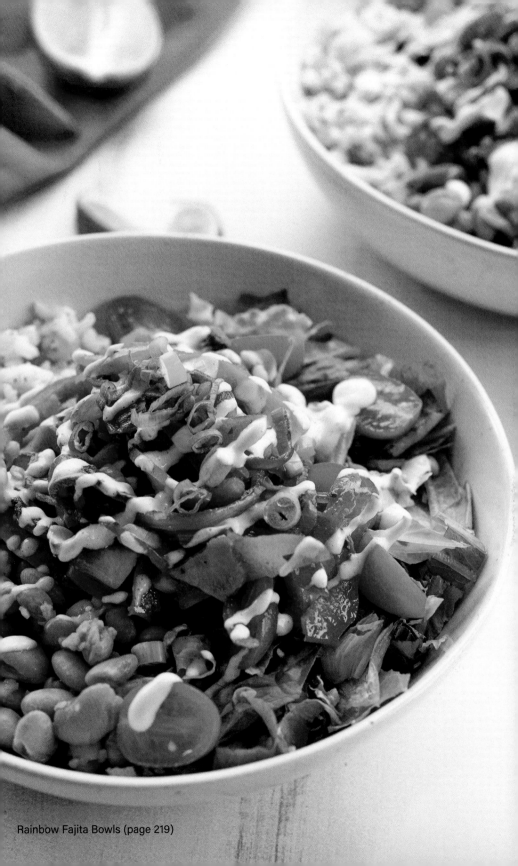

Rainbow Fajita Bowls (page 219)

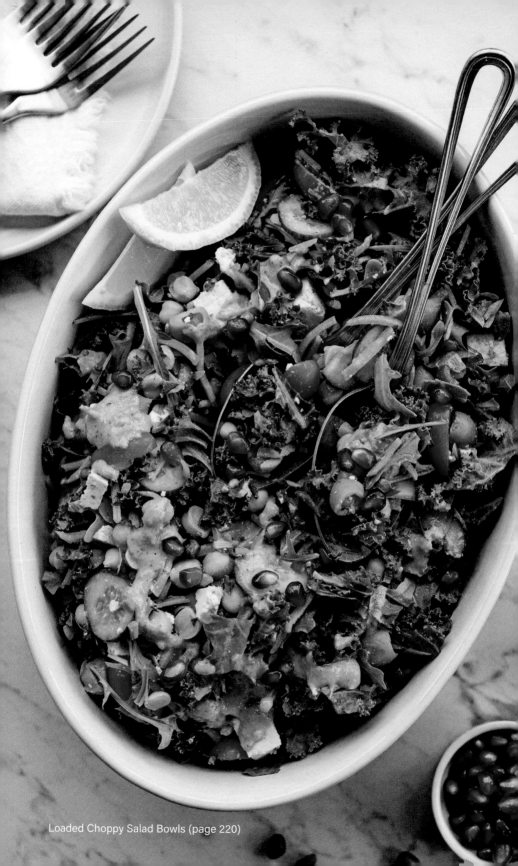

Loaded Choppy Salad Bowls (page 220)

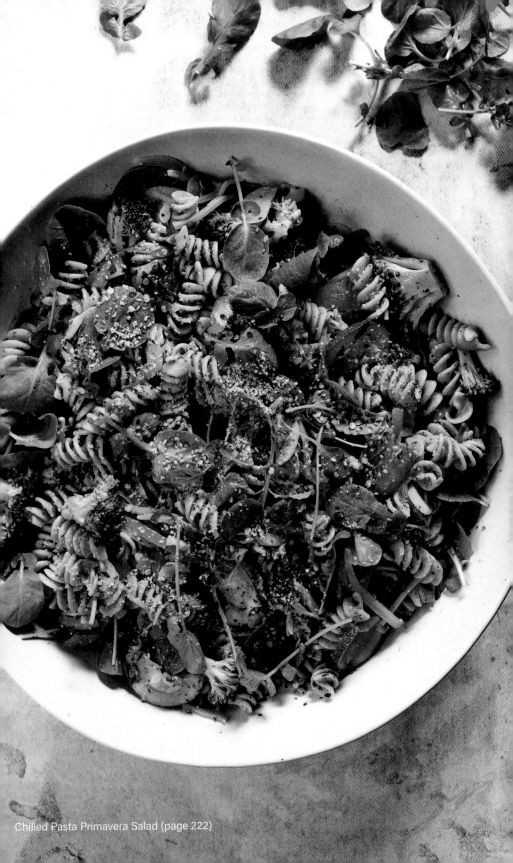

Chilled Pasta Primavera Salad (page 222)

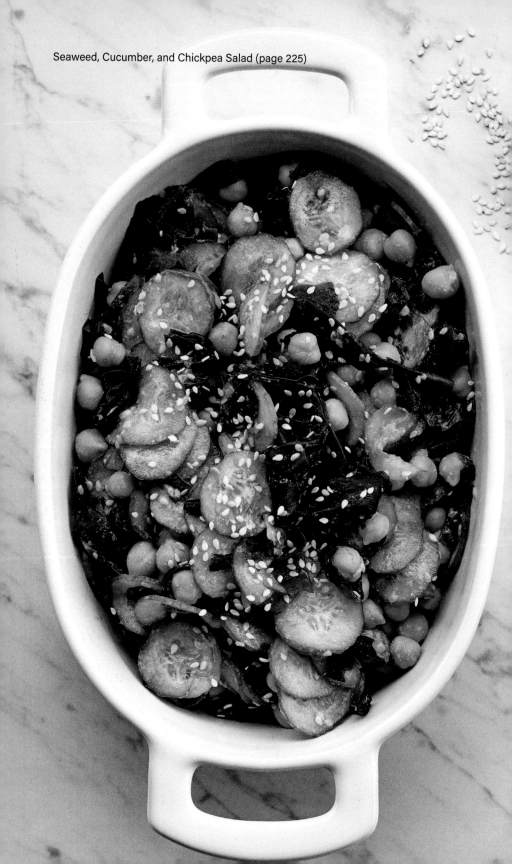

Seaweed, Cucumber, and Chickpea Salad (page 225)

is high in what is called *saturated* fat—the solid fat that raises cholesterol levels and is linked to loss of cognitive function in later life, among other health problems. Dairy products are even more densely packed with saturated fat, which is what imparts the gooey texture to cheese and butter.

When it comes to weight loss, animal products do not have the healthful fiber you need to tame your appetite. Nor do they have complex carbohydrate or other nutrients your body needs. As a group, people who avoid animal products are much slimmer than people who include it in their routines.

"Wait a minute," I hear you say. "Sure, beef isn't so good for you, but how about chicken or fish? Fish has good fats, right?"

The fact is, chicken is basically a lighter shade of beef. A small serving (100 grams) of "lean" roast beef has 3.4 grams of saturated ("bad") fat and 83 milligrams of cholesterol. For chicken, the numbers are 3.8 grams of saturated fat and 88 milligrams of cholesterol. Take off the skin, and you are still left with 2 grams of saturated fat and 89 milligrams of cholesterol (per 100 grams), with no fiber at all.

For fish, here are the numbers: Atlantic salmon is about 40 percent fat as a percentage of calories. Chinook salmon is over 50 percent. Most of that fat is not "good" fat. It is a mixture of saturated fats and other fats that you do not need at all.

In contrast, beans, vegetables, fruits, and grains have no cholesterol and virtually no saturated fat, but plenty of healthy fiber and complex carbohydrate.

Bottom line: It is better to get your protein from plants, and it is easy to do.

Cheese and Other Dairy Products

Cheese is addicting. Many people love it. But I am sorry to say cheese does not love you back. From a weight-control standpoint, dairy products will do you no favors. The number one nutrient in milk is sugar—lactose sugar. The number two nutrient is fat. And that makes sense, since milk's job is to fatten a growing calf. Condensing it into cheese concentrates the calories even more. If you were to send a slice of cheddar to a laboratory, you would learn that it is about 70 percent fat—mostly saturated fat. The average American consumes about *70,000 calories'* worth of cheese every year.

Cheese also has more sodium, ounce for ounce, than potato chips. A two-ounce serving of chips has 330 milligrams of sodium. Two ounces of cheddar have 350. For Edam, it's 500; and a two-ounce serving of Velveeta has 800. Think high blood pressure and water weight.

Cheese has something else that might surprise you. Dairy products contain *estradiol* and other female sex hormones (estrogens) that come from the cow. Dairy cows are artificially inseminated every year and are milked during much of their pregnancies, as their bodies are creating more and more estradiol. The hormones dribble down the milk-machine tubes, into your cheese sandwich, and eventually into your bloodstream.

Researchers believe that the estradiol in milk may be the reason why milk-drinking is linked to breast cancer. In China, milk is not a traditional part of the diet. Needless to say, Beijing is not Switzerland. However, over the last generation or so, Westernization has brought more and more dairy products to Asia. In 2004, researchers with the China Kadoorie Biobank study began tracking dairy intake in a large group of volunteers. Although only about 20 percent of women were drinking milk regularly, over the next decade, a clear-cut relationship emerged. For every small serving (50 grams, or about a fifth of a cup) of dairy products consumed daily, breast cancer risk jumped 19 percent.[4] So, a cup of dairy products a day would mean roughly a doubling of breast cancer risk.

In the United States, where dairy consumption is more universal and dairy products are added to many processed foods, it has been hard to compare large groups of women who avoid milk with those consuming larger amounts of it. However, in 2020, researchers at the Adventist Health Study-2 came out with stunning data. They took advantage of the fact that among Seventh-Day Adventists, a notably health-conscious religious group, there is a wide variation in dairy consumption and many people who avoid dairy products completely. Examining the diets and health of tens of thousands of women, the same pattern found in China became clear in this US-based population. High dairy users turned out to be 50 percent more likely to develop breast cancer, compared with those who generally avoided dairy products. Once again, the likely suspect was the female sex hormones in the dairy products.[5] Evidence also strongly links dairy products to prostate and ovarian cancer.

What about nonfat milk? Well, skimming the fat off is a good idea. But what you are left with is mostly sugar (lactose), with some dairy protein, which you already know you don't want, and, yes, estrogens. The concerns about cancer risk still apply. In fact, in Harvard's Physicians Health Study, the strongest associations between dairy intake and prostate cancer risk were for skim milk.[6]

What about yogurt? Yogurt is a dairy product with bacteria added. It has all the same problems of other dairy products—high in sugar and fat (unless the fat is removed), with traces of estrogens. And despite vigorous marketing of the value of "probiotics" (the commercially successful euphemism for bacteria), the added bacterial cultures have little, if any, actual health benefit. You have plenty of bacteria in your intestinal tract already, and these added traces are tiny by comparison. Moreover, what really counts for maintaining healthy gut bacteria is *everything else you eat*. In the same way that seeds grow in healthy soil, healthful bacteria flourish if your diet is rich in fiber from vegetables, fruits, beans, and whole grains. On a meaty diet, degrading animal proteins fill your digestive tract with fermenting amino acids, along with bile acids that your body produces to absorb fats. In this environment, unhealthful bacteria can overgrow, and probiotic pills and yogurt cannot stop them.

This happens fast. Harvard researchers tested a plant-based diet and a meat-based diet in volunteers, finding that the two diets could dramatically alter gut bacteria within *five days*.[7] The point is that it's not the sprinkle of probiotics in yogurt (or in supplements) that matters; it's your overall diet. Healthy gut bacteria thrive in a healthy high-fiber diet. Meat and other animal products send bile acids and degrading proteins to the gut, fueling the growth of unhealthy bacteria.

Even if an antibiotic has wiped out your gut bacteria, yogurt and bacteria supplements are generally not a good way to replace them. Researchers have found that with a good diet, healthful gut bacteria will come back on their own, and probiotics usually do not help.

Eggs

Eggs are not helpful for your waistline. About two-thirds of their calories come from fat, which readily adds to body fat. And about a third of that fat is "bad fat," that is, artery-clogging saturated fat. There is no complex carbohydrate and no fiber.

Eggs raise cholesterol. Yes, there have been occasional news stories, mostly propelled by the egg industry, suggesting that eggs do not raise cholesterol. But the scientific evidence has been clear for decades. In the same way that sugar you eat passes into your bloodstream, cholesterol you eat passes into your blood, too, and eggs have more of it than just about any other food.

In 2019, our research team reviewed every study ever published on the relationship between eggs and cholesterol.[8] There were 153 studies in all, some funded by governmental bodies, others funded by industry, especially the American Egg Board, a federally authorized, industry-funded program designed to promote egg consumption. In the vast majority of studies, egg consumption was associated with increased cholesterol levels. However, industry-funded researchers tended to interpret their findings more generously. For example, in a 2014 study of college freshmen, adding two eggs daily at breakfast led to a 15 mg/dl rise in LDL-cholesterol ("bad cholesterol") in fourteen weeks. That is a big increase. However, researchers could not be sure that the finding was not simply due to chance. Rather than saying so, they reported that eggs had no effect on cholesterol levels.[9]

Bottom line, eggs are dense in calories and are likely to raise your cholesterol level. An egg is a great environment for a growing chick but not good for your waistline or your arteries.

Oils

From a health standpoint, vegetable oils are much better than animal fats. They tend not to raise cholesterol levels. In fact, your body actually needs traces of the natural oils found in vegetables, fruits, and beans. The two essential fats your body needs are called *alpha-linolenic acid* and *linoleic acid* (this will not be on the test). You need only traces—these fats need to make up just 2 or 3 percent of your daily calories—and you will get them automatically in vegetables, fruits, and beans.

There is no need to add extra fat. If you add oil—cooking in it or slathering it on your foods—it will slow your weight loss. That is because all fats have 9 calories per gram. That is true of animal fats, and also true of vegetable oils. So the fryer grease cooked into French fries and the olive oil drenching your salad are packed with calories. A very few plant-derived foods are oily, too—nuts, seeds, and avocados. And yes, their fat has 9 calories per gram.

Think about this: You could eat an olive, or maybe two or three. Each one has only a trace of fat, and I would bet you've never eaten more than, say, a dozen at a sitting. However, oil companies extract the oil and discard the pulp and fiber, turning olives into something Mother Nature never envisioned—the oil of 5,000 to 8,000 olives crammed into a bottle.

For avoiding unwanted calories, it really does pay to avoid

cooking with oil. Instead, sauté in vegetable broth or water, use a nonstick pan, or favor steaming, baking, or roasting over typical frying. While you are at it, replacing oily salad dressings with flavorful vinegars or a squirt of lemon juice is a great idea, too.

Some people like to supplement with other natural oils, called EPA and DHA, in hopes of improving brain health. If you choose to do that, you will find plant-derived (vegan) EPA and DHA supplements online, without the extra fats that make fish fattening.

Mediterranean Diets

Perhaps surprisingly, Mediterranean diets do not work very well for weight loss. Yes, these diets sound romantic. Who would not want to sip a glass of wine at sunset on the coast of Tuscany? And because they include plenty of vegetables, Mediterranean diets may be healthier than what many people are eating. But they still contain enough fish, poultry, olive oil, some dairy, and other things, to pack in a lot of calories.

The term "Mediterranean diet" was coined by University of Minnesota researcher Ancel Keys in the 1950s, based on the dietary pattern of southern Italy. Vegetables, fruits, pasta, chickpeas, and other simple foods were everyday staples, and fish and poultry were commonplace, if not abundant. Wine was often served at mealtime. Dairy products and red meat were less common. For cooking, olive oil was preferred. Some studies have shown that this diet has an edge over a more typical American diet when it comes to heart health.

Our research team tested it out for its effects on weight. We invited sixty-two people who wanted to lose weight to join a study. Half were assigned to try a Mediterranean diet for sixteen weeks. The other half began a low-fat vegan diet for the same time period. After sixteen weeks, everyone took a break for four weeks, then switched to the opposite diet. So the Mediterranean group began the vegan diet and vice versa. In other words, everyone had a chance to try out both diets and compare them.

At first, the participants beginning the Mediterranean diet were eager to try this indulgent-seeming way of eating. But they soon started to complain. "Nothing is happening. When will I start to lose weight?" they asked. After sixteen weeks, they had lost essentially nothing. On the vegan diet, the results were very different. Participants were a bit nervous at first, wondering how they would like it. But soon they discovered the wide range of tastes available to them, and weight loss was rapid, as you might have guessed.

Then they switched. The Mediterranean group now started the vegan diet, finding that weight loss suddenly started to kick in. Meanwhile, the vegan group switched to a Mediterranean diet. To their dismay, they found the pounds piling back on rapidly. Many were angry, feeling that the Mediterranean diet is overhyped and ineffective. In the end, the Mediterranean diet led to no net weight loss at all, while on the vegan diet the average person lost thirteen pounds in sixteen weeks.[10]

Avocados

Avocados originated in Mexico and have been cultivated for thousands of years. They are delicious. But by a quirk of nature, the avocado tree packs a lot of fat into its fruit. That is why people smear avocados onto toast like butter.

A typical avocado has about 20 grams of fat,[11] and, as you know, every gram packs 9 calories. For comparison, look at other fruits: A typical apple has less than a gram of fat (0.2 grams, to be exact). An orange is about the same. That is why an avocado has three times more calories than an apple or an orange (230 versus about 75 for an apple and 70 for an orange). Think of it as a nut pretending to be a fruit.

In its defense, the fat in an avocado is not the same as in butter or chicken fat. About 60 percent of the fat is *monounsatured* fat, the kind that also predominates in olive oil and tends not to raise cholesterol. About 14 percent is saturated ("bad") fat, the kind that does raise cholesterol and is linked to Alzheimer's disease. That is much less than in animal fats. An avocado also carries about 9 grams of fiber, unlike cheese and butter, which have no fiber at all.

The avocado industry has been eager to show that, despite their load of fat and calories, avocados are good for you. The Avocado Nutrition Center launched a huge study, called the Habitual Diet and Avocado Trial (HAT). It recruited 1,008 overweight volunteers, giving half of them free avocados and encouraging them to have one daily, and asking the other half to continue their usual, mostly avocado-free diets.

Their hypothesis was that avocados would reduce *visceral* fat— that is, the fat that accumulates around the intestines and other organs. It did not work out that way. Three months into the study, the avocado group had not lost weight at all. On average, the participants had gained a bit of weight, slightly more than the non-avocado group. By six months, both groups leveled off. Neither group lost weight, and they had slightly more visceral fat than before.[12]

If you are eating a typical American diet, avocados are not necessarily more fattening than many of the other foods you are eating. However, if you are modifying your food choices to lose weight, they are among the foods that are likely to slow your progress. Does this mean you should never have an avocado? There is no need to say "never." But when you are on a weight-loss trajectory, you might want to set them aside for the moment.

Coconut and Palm Oils

Coconut and palm oils deserve their own special condemnatory section. Food writers love their gooey mouth feel, and manufacturers promote them as healthful. You will find them added to all manner of foods, from peanut butter to vegan cheeses, to create a creamy texture.

Healthy they are not. For starters, they have 9 calories per gram, like chicken fat, olive oil, and every other fat or oil. But the *type* of fat they harbor is a problem. Unlike corn oil, olive oil, and other vegetable oils, they are very high in *saturated* fat.

As a result of all that "bad fat," their effect on cholesterol is not much different from that of animal fats. In 2020, a meta-analysis of sixteen research studies summed up the findings on coconut oil: It clearly raises levels of "bad cholesterol," that is, LDL cholesterol, in your bloodstream.[13] Think "heart attack" and "Alzheimer's disease." The verdict on palm oil was already in. In 2015, researchers concluded that, like coconut oil, it raises bad cholesterol.[14] In addition, saturated fat interferes with the production of GLP-1, an appetite-taming hormone we will discuss in the next chapter.

So, slick back your hair with coconut oil. Shine your shoes with it. Polish your car. Make a candle. But don't eat it, and don't buy foods that use it as an ingredient. It is fattening and unhealthy.

Gluten-Free Foods

As we saw in chapter 2, if you are one of the not quite 1 percent of the population with celiac disease—a severe reaction to the gluten protein in wheat, barley, rye, and a few other foods—avoiding gluten is a must.[15] And perhaps one in ten people find that avoiding gluten improves their digestion or makes them feel better mentally. But for everyone else, avoiding gluten brings no reward at all. If you are avoiding pasta, bread, et cetera, you are depriving yourself of healthful foods for no reason.

It should be said that most foods are gluten-free anyway. Fruits, vegetables, and beans never had it, and neither do most grains, such as rice, corn, quinoa, or millet.

Artificial Sweeteners

In the United States, a variety of artificial sweeteners have been approved for sale by the Food and Drug Administration—saccharin

(Sweet'n Low), aspartame (Equal, NutraSweet), and sucralose (Splenda), among others. For the most part, they do not appear to be dangerous.

However, they do not help much. If you are replacing sugar, you are replacing one of the lowest-calorie foods you are eating. As you know by now, sugar has only 4 calories per gram, while fats and oils have more than double that—9 calories per gram. So if you ate a ham and cheese sandwich with a Diet Coke instead of a regular Coke, you would have been better off replacing the contents of the sandwich.

Replacing sugar with artificial sweeteners does not prevent diabetes, either. Researchers have found that, overall, the amount of sugar you eat is not associated with your risk of developing diabetes.[16] This may be a revelation to those who thought that diabetes is caused by sugar. Type 2 diabetes actually starts as a condition called *insulin resistance,* which comes from the buildup of fat particles in your muscle and liver cells that interfere with insulin's ability to work. This discovery led the way to the development of diets that remove that fat buildup and can greatly improve and sometimes even eliminate diabetes. If you would like more information on this, please have a look at my book *Dr. Neal Barnard's Program for Reversing Diabetes.*

This is not to say that sugar is innocuous. Sugar lures us to cookies and cakes, which often contain a load of butter, shortening, or oil that pack in the calories. Also, artificial sweeteners maintain the desire for sugar, and may heighten it. If that persistent sugar craving leads you to eat more cookies, cakes, and pastries in general, their fatty ingredients will add to weight issues.

Although most artificial sweeteners do not seem to be dangerous, researchers at the Cleveland Clinic made a troubling finding about one common sweetener, erythritol. Studying a large group of heart patients, they noticed that those with higher blood levels of erythritol were more likely to have a heart attack or stroke or to die within the next three years. The researchers found that the sweetener makes blood platelets more likely to clump together, forming a life-threatening clot. This was bad news, because erythritol is in a large array of sugar-free products. It does not take a huge dose, apparently. The amounts used in diet products are likely more than enough to cause the problem.[17]

For natural sweetness, fruits are nature's pick. Speaking of which, date sugar is just ground-up dates—it's the whole fruit, as a powder. Stevia is a natural plant extract that adds a sweet taste to recipes. Used in modest amounts it appears to be safe.

Alcohol

Some people have suggested that moderate drinking might have benefits. An occasional glass of wine might be good for the heart was the idea. Some studies have also suggested that, in modest doses, wine might reduce the risk of developing Alzheimer's disease. In 2022, researchers compiled the evidence from nine different countries and suggested that people who consumed an occasional glass of wine had about 28 percent less risk of developing Alzheimer's disease, compared with their teetotaling friends.[18]

However, in April 2023 the party hats all fell off when the American Medical Association published a new analysis of the evidence. They found that previous studies classified many people as teetotalers who in fact were people who'd had health problems that forced them to stop drinking. Compared with these not so healthy people, modest drinkers had an advantage. But in a more careful analysis comparing people who were generally similar in all respects apart from their alcohol use, the seeming benefits of modest drinking vanished. There was no significant benefit from having an occasional drink or from daily modest use. Above that level, it was clear that the more people drink, the more likely they are to die.[19]

Health authorities often recommend that women have no more than 20 grams of alcohol per day, which means seven ounces (200 milliliters) of wine, sixteen ounces (475 milliliters) of regular beer, or one ounce (30 milliliters) of liquor. For men, typical limits are 30 grams of alcohol, which means ten ounces (300 milliliters) of wine, twenty-four ounces (720 milliliters) of regular beer, or two ounces (60 milliliters) of liquor. However, even one drink per day increases a woman's risk of breast cancer. Alcohol is also linked to colon cancer and other forms of the disease, as well as liver disease, accidents, and ruined lives. And there are better ways to reduce the risk of dementia. When people avoid "bad" fats and other risky exposures (e.g., aluminum or excessive iron or copper), exercise regularly, and follow a vegan diet, it is not clear that alcohol adds anything beneficial.

That said, a glass of red wine does contain healthy bioactive compounds, including resveratrol, phenolic acids, and flavonoids. But you can get the same from the grapes themselves, needless to say. Indeed, grape juice—without the alcohol—seems to have helpful cognitive effects.[20] The same appears to be true for blueberries, as we saw in chapter 2.[21]

If It's Bad for You, Throw It Out

Dr. Steven Lome is a cardiologist in Monterey, California, and an accomplished runner. In November 2022, he was about three miles into a half-marathon when, directly in front of him, another runner suddenly collapsed. He was pulseless and not breathing. Dr. Lome immediately began CPR, and other runners came to help and called 911. Eventually, a defibrillator arrived. Despite having a deadly heart rhythm called ventricular fibrillation, the man's heart responded, and an ambulance carried him to the hospital where, miraculously, he recovered.

Needless to say, this was not a normal race. But with the man in good hands, Dr. Lome decided to finish his race. It was a good thing he did because, just as he arrived at the finish line, a second man collapsed in front of him. He, too, was pulseless and not breathing. Again, Dr. Lome administered CPR and, when a defibrillator arrived, he was able to restart the man's heart. He survived, too.

The extraordinary day became a focus for newspaper and television stories everywhere. The Today show reunited Dr. Lome with the grateful men, both of whom had decided to make big diet changes at Dr. Lome's urging.

Perhaps the most remarkable part of the story, however, is that Dr. Lome had had an amazing recovery of his own. Growing up in the Chicago suburbs, his family gave little thought to the risks of unhealthy foods. His parents struggled with serious weight problems, along with diabetes and other issues. He himself began gaining weight early on, and things worsened in medical school and residency.

In his medical training, nutrition was a neglected topic, and many of his mentors followed poor diets. He recalls asking one of his professors about how best to help a patient with diabetes, and the professor, who was seriously overweight himself, told him, "The only thing I know about diabetes is that I have it."

On his commute to the hospital each morning, Dr. Lome had a habit of stopping at Starbucks or Dunkin' Donuts for a sausage and egg sandwich and plenty of coffee to recover from the rocky night's sleep that resulted from sleep apnea, a common consequence of obesity. He had high blood pressure, cholesterol problems, back pain, and acid reflux.

Apart from his personal health problems, as a cardiologist,

he was frustrated. He was prescribing medications and other treatments as he was trained to do, but for many patients, heart problems continued.

He decided he needed to find a better way to eat. He turned to the US government's official nutrition guidance, called the Dietary Guidelines for Americans, and resolved to follow it. He shifted his diet from red meat to chicken and fish, with oil in moderation. He cut down on cookies, doughnuts, and other snack foods. He also began to exercise seriously. At 260 pounds, he signed up for a marathon. The training was grueling, as was the race itself, but he managed to finish. And yet despite everything, he was still overweight with high cholesterol.

After struggling for two years with what was supposed to be a healthy diet and exercise program, he saw a film called *Forks over Knives*. It profiled health experts—T. Colin Campbell, PhD, and Caldwell Esselstyn, MD—who called for throwing out animal products altogether and focusing instead on healthful plant-based foods. They laid out compelling evidence. And he realized they were right. He had thought he needed meat for protein, that eggs were good for him, and that moderating his diet ought to help, and now he was convinced that path was a mistake. He resolved to try the approach discussed in the film.

After a week he could see his life being transformed. His weight gradually dropped to 170 pounds, which at six-foot-one put him well into the healthy weight range. His cholesterol normalized, too. He signed up for more marathons, finding his pace improved dramatically. While chicken, fish, and moderation did not work, throwing out unhealthy foods did. "We don't have cigarettes in moderation, why should we have unhealthy foods in moderation?" he asks.

His father was inspired by his example and adopted the same diet. He lost more than one hundred pounds and got off all his medications. His mother did the same thing, and her diabetes disappeared.

Dr. Lome's wife, Helen, is a doctor as well, specializing in family medicine. Together, they have guided their children to a healthy plant-based diet and are delighted that they have a measure of protection against the problems so many families struggle with.

So, we have learned that the not-so-good-for-you foods include meat, dairy products, eggs, oils, artificial sweeteners, and alcohol. And, of course, it pays to have your foods in as simple and natural a form as possible. Now you are an expert in which foods are healthful and which foods do more harm than good. In chapter 5, we will start building our meals.

CHAPTER 4

Drugs and Money

Before moving on, let's have a word about weight-loss drugs. Over the years, they have been very popular and often controversial, and most have been withdrawn from the market due to side effects, as you will learn below. Among the newer drugs is semaglutide, which is marketed as Ozempic for diabetes and as Wegovy for weight loss. Both are weekly injectables that reduce appetite and, for people with diabetes, reduce blood sugar. Doctors call them *GLP-1 receptor agonists*. I'll explain the technical terms more below.

Their manufacturer, Novo Nordisk, is promoting them wildly with advertisements, payments to physicians, sponsorships of medical organizations, and intense lobbying. The media buzz has no doubt caught your attention, and you may be asking, "Should I take a weight-loss drug?" Hold that thought.

Jasmine

Jasmine was thirty-eight when she decided she'd had enough. She had started gaining weight in junior high, and at her high school graduation, she was about forty pounds heavier than she wanted to be. Her family was concerned because her blood pressure and blood sugar were creeping upward, too.

At first, she tried to just not eat. For an entire day, she refused food. The starvation days led to binge days, leaving her feeling discouraged and out of control. Food was sometimes her friend and other times felt like her worst enemy.

Her parents brought her to a dietitian, who prescribed an eating plan that strictly limited her portions and calories, but after a day or two, she found it impossible to follow. She was told to exercise, which she did, but it did not affect her weight very much. Other diet attempts followed.

Fast-forward two decades. After reading a news article about Wegovy, Jasmine found a doctor who was willing to prescribe it. The doctor explained that since her parents were overweight, too, and her diets had not worked, she probably had a genetic problem. Hopefully the injections would help. Her insurance did not cover the cost, so she filled the prescription at her own expense, well over a thousand dollars per month. The first several weeks were rough, with nausea and diarrhea. But the symptoms gradually subsided. The weight loss was certainly noticeable but was not as dramatic as she had hoped. Eventually, she decided to stop the expensive injections to see if she could maintain without them. But within a few months, the weight she had lost had come back.

At that point, she contacted a medical center specializing in nutrition where, for the first time, she learned about the foods that could help her lose weight over the long term. She decided to try a plant-based diet. She met a dietitian who helped her plan a menu that, to her surprise, had no portion limits at all. Nonetheless, it worked surprisingly quickly. Over time, she lost a great deal of weight, and her blood sugar and blood pressure normalized, too. She told her parents about what she was doing. Although they were in their sixties and had more or less given up on their weight issues, they decided to try it as well, and lost a substantial amount of weight, too.

Jasmine came to believe that her problem was not genetic but was instead related to food habits she had shared with her parents, and that getting on a better path could help all of them.

So, back to our question: Should you take a weight-loss drug? The answer for the vast majority of people is no—there are much better, safer, and more long-lasting ways to trim away unwanted weight. This does not rule out their use in unusual situations, but let me explain the issues.

A Checkered History

In the 1930s, amphetamines were commonly used and are still marketed (legitimately) for attention deficit hyperactivity disorder. But their use for weight loss has run aground due to a wide range of physical and psychological side effects and a tendency to become habit-forming.

In the 1990s, "fen-phen" became wildly popular. That was the short name for a combination drug (phentermine and fenfluramine) that was soon pulled from the market because it damaged heart valves with potentially fatal consequences.

Lorcaserin, sold under the brand name Belviq, was a commercially successful appetite-reducer until it was withdrawn in 2020 due to cancer risks. Many other drugs have come and gone as their risks have become known.

Others remain on the market. Apart from semaglutide, the US

Food and Drug Administration has approved several other weight-loss drugs:

- Liraglutide (Saxenda, Victoza) is similar to semaglutide. It is marketed mainly for diabetes but also has an appetite-reducing effect.
- Naltrexone/bupropion (Contrave) combines an opiate-blocker (naltrexone) with an antidepressant (bupropion). It reduces appetite.
- Phentermine (Adipex-P, Lomaira) is used to suppress appetite. It is also prescribed in combination with topiramate under the brand name Qsymia, and causes modest weight loss.
- Orlistat (Xenical, Alli) is a nonprescription drug that blocks the absorption of fat from the digestive tract. The idea is that you eat the chicken wings, and the grease ends up in the toilet. Gastrointestinal side effects are common, and weight loss is modest.
- Setmelanotide (Imcivree) is prescribed for rare genetic disorders.

In addition, the diabetes drug tirzepatide, marketed as Mounjaro, also causes weight loss, similar to semaglutide.

Ozempic and Wegovy cause only modest weight loss over the short term.[1] However, in obese adults participating in longer research studies, it has been common to observe significant weight loss, which, in turn, ought to reduce obesity's health consequences.[2] However, weight loss typically seems to plateau well before individuals reach a healthy weight.

These drugs have adverse effects: nausea, vomiting, diarrhea, gastroesophageal reflux, and, more rarely, gallbladder disease and pancreatitis. In a French study, drugs of this type were linked to a 58 percent increased risk of thyroid cancer.[3] Because of concerns about the possibility of harm to a fetus, they are generally contraindicated for women who are or may become pregnant.

In the United States, Wegovy currently costs about $1,600 per month ($1,300 with manufacturer coupons). Elsewhere, the price varies greatly from country to country. Here is the problem: If you stop taking the drug, most of the lost weight returns. In Novo Nordisk's research, among people who lost 39.8 pounds taking the drug, stopping the drug was followed by a regain of more than 25 pounds.[4]

So the idea is, once you have started it, you continue on it for the rest of your life. Taking semaglutide is like having a subscription to a weight-loss service that packs up and leaves if you stop paying.

Most people do indeed stop. In a 2020 US study of 4,791 people taking semaglutide for diabetes, 48 percent quit taking the drug in the first year, and 70 percent stopped within two years.[5] In a 2022 UK study including 589 users, 45 percent stopped within one year, and 65 percent stopped within two years.[6]

A 2023 report was even worse. Conducted by Prime Therapeutics, a pharmacy benefits manager owned by Blue Cross Blue Shield plans and focusing on people using semaglutide and similar drugs to lose weight, the report found that more than two-thirds of users quit within a year.[7]

Why stop the drug? Side effects, expense, annoyance at having to inject the drug, and results that did not measure up to expectations (most users do not achieve results that match those found in research trials[8])—or to what can be achieved by effective diet changes.

Needless to say, insurance companies do not want to pay for it: Of the 260 million adults in the United States, more than one-third are obese. If just one in ten obese Americans used Wegovy, the cost would approach $150 billion per year. Prime Therapeutics found that in a sample of individuals starting these drugs for weight loss, insurance costs averaged $13,048 per year before beginning the injections and increased to $25,850 per year after starting treatment. An increase in the use of these drugs by just 1 percent of an insured population was estimated to add $14.50 per member per month to self-insured employers' insurance costs.[9]

Why are the drugs so expensive? The price does not reflect the cost of making the drug. Rather, this figure is padded to increase company profits. It also includes marketing expenses. Novo Nordisk spends millions on advertising and pays American doctors about $27 million each year in speaking and consulting fees. Its political action committee contributes to politicians' campaign funds. During the 2021–2022 election cycle, Novo Nordisk's PAC donated $287,250 to federal candidates, including hefty donations to the campaigns of cosponsors of a bill that would require the federal government to pay for Novo Nordisk's drugs.

On January 1, 2023, CBS's popular television program *60 Minutes* ran a thirteen-minute story about Wegovy. It looked like an ordinary news story. The host, Leslie Stahl, interviewed two medical experts who praised the drug. In fact, they praised it a little too much. As the program went along, it started to smell like an advertisement. Indeed, it turned out that Novo Nordisk was a *60 Minutes* sponsor, and both medical experts were paid Novo Nordisk consultants. The US government's Open Payments website shows that, between 2015 and 2021, the two doctors had received $100,284 from Novo Nordisk, and about three times that amount from drug companies overall.

The program was, in fact, effectively an advertisement, and should have been presented as such. My organization, the Physicians Committee, called foul and asked the Food and Drug Administration to investigate how a promotional advertisement had been disguised as a news story.

And Here Is the Surprise

Surprisingly enough, these drugs do artificially what your body can do naturally.

When you eat food, your digestive tract releases a natural compound called GLP-1 into your bloodstream (GLP-1 stands for glucagon-like peptide-1). GLP-1 is like a switch that turns down your appetite. This is part of how your body regulates eating. You feel hungry, so you have something to eat. Then, as the meal begins, your body releases GLP-1, which travels to your brain and signals you to stop eating. Your body makes GLP-1 as you eat breakfast, again during lunch, and again at dinner. It is your appetite off switch.

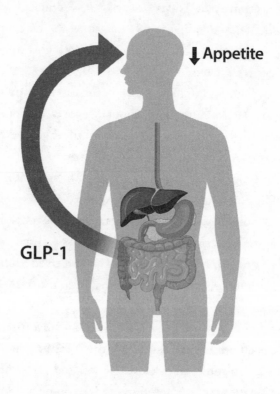

Ozempic and Wegovy are synthetic drugs that stimulate the body's receptors for GLP-1. In other words, they are doing essentially the same thing that food is supposed to do. Because they are injections, they can push the effect higher than nature would have done.

So if our body has a natural GLP-1 system, why is it not working? Why do so many of us feel hungry all the time and gain weight?

Novo Nordisk would like you to believe that you have a genetic problem that is driving your appetite. Maybe, but not likely.

The fact is that the GLP-1 system was programmed into the human body long ago, and the foods that activate it best are those rich in fiber and carbohydrates.[10] There were no dairy products at all until about ten thousand years ago, so the 70,000 calories' worth of cheese an average American eats each year nowadays was nowhere in sight. There were no slaughterhouses producing the one million chickens Americans eat every hour. There were no candy factories or fast-food drive-throughs. It turns out that high-fat, high-calorie foods like cheese, meat, and chocolate do not activate our GLP-1 system very well. Similarly, saturated fats (found in dairy products and meat, for example) are not so good at GLP-1 release, while unsaturated fats (found in plants) do a better job.

Our appetite-control system is not working because we are not eating the high-fiber, high-complex carbohydrate foods that activate it. Instead, we are eating meat, cheese, and greasy foods that do not activate our appetite-control system very well.

If butter is not good for turning on our GLP-1 appetite-control system, but foods like beans, whole grains, and starchy vegetables that are rich in fiber and complex carbohydrates work much better, a diet shift ought to boost GLP-1 naturally—without any sort of injection at all. My research colleague, Hana Kahleova, and her team put this idea to the test. In fifty people with type 2 diabetes, they tested two different sandwiches. They held exactly the same number of calories, but one was plant-based and the other was meat-based. The participants ate one of the sandwiches, and the researchers took blood tests to see if GLP-1 levels increased. Later, they tested the other sandwich.

The results were dramatic. The plant-based sandwich increased GLP-1 secretion more than twofold, compared with the meat sandwich.[11] Further research confirmed the findings.[12, 13]

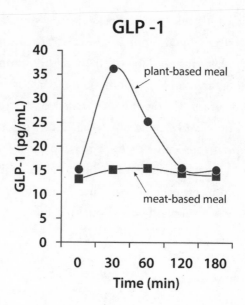

By now you may be asking, "If the right foods stimulate GLP-1 naturally, why would anyone want Wegovy with all its expense, side effects, and weight regain when you stop the injections?"

The reason is that no one told them. Drug companies tell you what suits their sales promotions, and they pay doctors to discuss their products at their hospitals and medical schools. Novo Nordisk is not about to tell you that a diet high in fiber and complex carbohydrate will activate your GLP-1 system naturally.

In its defense, Novo Nordisk might say that doctors are supposed to prescribe semaglutide only for patients for whom diet changes did not work. But that raises the question, what sort of diet had they been given? If a "diet" means trying to starve the weight off by restricting calories, it is hard for *anyone* to sustain. Likewise, a Mediterranean diet sounds healthy, but it does not cause weight loss. More or less *everyone* who tries to lose weight with these methods ends up disappointed. The answer is not an expensive injectable; the answer is solid information and support for changing your eating habits in a healthier direction.

Regrettably, doctors often give faulty advice—or no advice at all—when it comes to nutrition. A recent survey of internal medicine residents revealed that a majority had had little or no nutrition training.[14] But they know all about prescription drugs. The pharmaceutical manufacturers make sure of it. The Physicians Committee is working hard to improve medical knowledge, providing comprehensive nutrition information for medical trainees and physicians in practice.

Other medicines can affect your weight, too. Let us have a look at two particularly common ones.

Cholesterol-Lowering Medications

Many medications cause weight gain. Among the most surprising are cholesterol-lowering drugs. Atorvastatin (Lipitor), simvastatin (Zocor), rosuvastatin (Crestor), and other statin drugs are big sellers. But it turns out they can boost your appetite, leading you to eat more than you otherwise would.

Here's what is going on: Normally, if you gain weight, your body's fat cells release a hormone called *leptin,* which enters your bloodstream and reduces your appetite. The more leptin you produce, the better appetite control you have, at least in theory. However, statin drugs used for cholesterol control have the unfortunate effect of reducing your body's ability to produce leptin.[15] With less leptin in your bloodstream, your appetite ramps up.

Researchers at the Mayo Clinic in Rochester, Minnesota, tested these drugs in cultures of human fat cells. The more they applied statin drugs to the fat cells, the more they blocked the cells' ability to make leptin.

The effects show up on the scale. In a 2015 review combining the results of twelve prior studies, cholesterol-lowering statin drugs were indeed associated with weight gain.[16] They also increased the risk of developing diabetes, something also seen in other studies.[17]

These effects are not huge, but they are pushing your health in the wrong direction. Researchers are also concerned about something else. It appears that many patients imagine that if they take a statin drug, it is no longer necessary to think about their eating habits. In fact, I was once dining with a group of doctors, one of whom dug into a steak while saying, "It's okay, I'm on Lipitor." He was only half kidding.

Researchers tracked the food intake of participants in the National Health and Nutrition Examination Survey over a decade.[18] In 1999 to 2000, statin users seemed relatively health-conscious, limiting their fat and calorie intake, presumably in response to medical advice. As the years went by, however, statin users seemed to be paying less and less attention to what they were eating. By 2010, they were eating more fat and more calories than people who were not using statins. The researchers suggested that statins may give the patients—or their doctors—a false sense of security, leading them to be more indulgent than they would otherwise be. Their conclusion: "We believe that the goal of statin treatment, as with any pharmacotherapy, should be to allow patients to decrease risks that cannot be decreased without medication, not to empower them to put butter on their steaks."

That statement may seem a bit harsh. It may, in fact, be the patients' doctors who have allowed a more blasé attitude about diet, believing that as long as the patient is taking prescribed medication, the doctor's work is done.

Insulin

Insulin causes weight gain. If you are taking insulin for diabetes and you improve your eating habits so that you can reduce your dose or get off your insulin altogether, it becomes easier to lose weight.

The UK Prospective Diabetes Study tested the effects of intensive drug treatment for diabetes. The study included 3,867 people newly diagnosed with type 2 diabetes. The idea was to see if more intensive treatment with insulin or oral medications could reduce the risk of complications. Over the next decade, those in the intensive-treatment group using insulin gained about fifteen pounds.[19] Those treated intensively with oral medications gained extra weight, too, although not to the extent seen with insulin treatment.

In our research studies of people with type 2 diabetes who begin a low-fat, vegan diet, we see exactly the opposite. Most participants taking insulin are able to reduce or stop their insulin use. And they *lose* weight in the process.

A Note of Caution

There is an important role for medications. As powerful as diet changes can be, they are not perfect, either. So if you are taking medications, talk with your physician about the diet changes you are making and work with your doctor to adjust your doses or stop your medication if and when the time is right.

PART 2

LET'S GET STARTED

CHAPTER 5

Meal Planning for Breakfast, Lunch, Dinner, and Snacks

You are now an expert in power foods for weight loss and the best of health. So let's put that power to work. Incorporate these foods into your routine as much as you can. Use them to replace unhealthful foods that may be in your routine currently.

Instead of ordinary French toast, let's use the power-food toppings, like cinnamon, blueberries, and bananas, to turn that ordinary breakfast into one that helps you meet your health goals. Instead of bacon and eggs for breakfast, how about a big bowl of old-fashioned oatmeal topped with sliced strawberries? The more you plug in the power foods, the more benefit you get.

At some point soon, you will want to do a field trip to the grocery store and/or health food store, explore the aisles, and see what hidden gems you find. You will have lots of great discoveries. Take this approach with you to restaurants, too. Yes, most have the right foods if you know what to look for. In chapter 6, I'll share restaurant tips with you.

Be sure to share what you know with your family and friends. Everyone loves food, and everyone wants to be healthier.

Go for the Max

When you are ready, let me encourage you to take another step. In our research studies and at the Barnard Medical Center, we use a special technique to help people experience what is as close to a perfect diet as possible. For a three-week period, we kick out unhealthy foods completely and emphasize the power foods at every meal to maximize the results on the scale *now*. For many people, this short experiment is life-changing. In chapter 7, I will show you how you can do the same.

Great Meal Ideas

Let's start by looking at how the power foods turn into meals. They can be tweaks of your favorites or they could be new meal ideas. In the descriptions below and in the recipe section, you will find choices for three different scenarios, depending on the mood you are in:

- **Convenient.** If cooking is just not you, it is easier than ever to get food on the table without lighting up the stove. We will look at quick ways to do that.
- **Easy.** If you are comfortable in the kitchen and like to take charge of what goes into your meals, we will look at the treasury of quick and easy meals built from familiar ingredients.
- **Elegant.** If you are planning a special occasion, we will explore recipes that deliver health power in an upscale package.

As you review your options, I encourage you to make a list of the meal ideas that appeal to you. Take a piece of paper, and mark categories for breakfast, lunch, dinner, and snacks. Then, jot down foods that you feel will work for you. This will help you visualize your meals and will be handy when you shop for foods. Then, try them. If they turn out to be winners, keep them. If not, scratch them off your list.

Let's start with ridiculously easy breakfast ideas, focusing first on some everyday foods to see how simple tweaks can pump up their health power.

Breakfast

Cereals. Let's say your usual morning breakfast is a bowl of cereal. You shake the cornflakes into a bowl and add some milk and sugar. Quick and convenient, for sure. And cornflakes, oat cereals, wheat or rice cereals, and other simple grains are perfectly fine to the extent they retain their natural fiber and do not have a lot of added ingredients. But let's add some weight-loss power to this simple breakfast.

You may remember from chapter 2 that blueberries, strawberries, and their cousins get their color from anthocyanins, and that researchers have found that anthocyanin-rich foods are associated with reduced body fat. In fact, they are at the top of our list of power foods. So let's use them to top our cereal. Sliced bananas are great, too. They are appetite-tamers but are surprisingly modest in calories. Next time you're at the store, pick up these healthy toppings and add them to your cereal.

Next, let's rethink the milk. Cow's milk's main nutrient is sugar (lactose) and its number two nutrient is fat (unless you're using skim). We can do better than this. Right next to the cow's milk in the dairy case is soy milk, reminding us that Harvard researchers rated soy products among the top foods for weight-loss power, along with their other benefits described in chapter 2. If you prefer, other nondairy milks are fine, too (except for coconut milk, which is high in saturated fat).

Okay! You've just combined a healthy grain with plenty of power-food toppings and avoided unhealthful additions. If this healthy bowl of cereal sounds good, let's put it on your list.

Let's try another easy example. If your cooking skills include being able to boil water, let's try a bowl of hot oatmeal and take advantage of its appetite-taming soluble fiber. Instant is okay. But if you choose old-fashioned oats, you will find they cook nearly as fast and will keep you feeling full longer.

Next, toppings: We can top it with blueberries, raspberries, strawberries, sliced bananas, raisins, or whatever calls to you. And how about a sprinkle of cinnamon? As you will recall, scientists believe that its natural ingredient, *cinnamaldehyde*, tackles the appetite and also increases your calorie burn. In the recipe section, you will find some wonderful variations on morning oats, including one for people who feel a need for an extra protein punch.

For a lighter taste, you can do the same with Cream of Wheat. It cooks up fast and can be topped with anything you like. If you are from the American South, you might be partial to grits. They cook in no time. Tweak number one is to leave out the butter. Then choose whatever toppings you like for a sweet or savory breakfast. Have a look at the quick and easy recipes for Cajun Grits (page 181) or Cheesy Grits and "Bacon" (page 175). You will be amazed at how traditional flavors are incorporated into healthful foods.

If a bowl of hot oatmeal, Cream of Wheat, or grits with healthy toppings sounds appealing, let's add it to your list. If not, leave it off.

Okay, you've got the idea. We are taking simple, familiar items and tweaking them to put the power foods to work. Here are more breakfast ideas to explore:

Waffles and Pancakes. If waffles or pancakes are your thing, skip the butter, and check out the amazing twists on each of these in the recipe section. If we get this right, we will be taking advantage of healthful grains and weight-loss toppings, and our breakfasts will be delicious. Note that you can make pancakes from oats or other kinds of flour, too.

If you are going for convenience, you will find handy mixes and frozen waffles that let the toaster do the work. The Achilles' heel of waffles and pancakes is the array of fatty ingredients sometimes packed into them. Skip products with eggs and milk, and favor those lowest in fat. Next time you are at the store, take a few minutes to check out the frozen food aisle and read the labels. Popular brands of frozen waffles include Simple Truth (Kroger), 365 brand (Whole Foods), Kashi, Nature's Path, and Van's Foods, among many others.

And now for some power-food artistry. Think of a waffle or pancake as a blank canvas. Cinnamon, strawberries, raspberries, blueberries, and sliced bananas are your colors. Channel your inner Jackson Pollock.

French Toast. French toast is everyone's favorite. See the recipe section for the best French toast you have ever had—flavored with a trace of nutmeg and drizzled in cinnamon blueberry sauce. Time-wise, there is nothing to it. You just dip bread into the mix and plunk it in a nonstick pan. Like waffles and pancakes, the problems start with eggs, milk, and butter. But it is easy to steer clear of these fatty ingredients. And, by now, you know the power-food toppings.

EASY ELEGANCE

If you are hosting a brunch, French toast is quick and easy. And let's bring a touch of elegance with these easy additions:

- A substantial bread: a sliced baguette or sourdough bread
- A sprinkle of confectioners' sugar
- A mint leaf
- A selection of syrups: maple, blueberry, strawberry, hazelnut
- Fresh blueberries, strawberries, raspberries, blackberries, and cinnamon

Keep in mind, "elegance" often derives from including things that are just a bit unusual. So while a bowl of berries is good, three different berries is better, and kumquats are downright exotic, especially if they are still on their branches.

You might also order a fruit display from Edible Arrangements or a similar delivery service. It looks like a bouquet, but each "stem" is a piece of fruit, including plenty of power foods, like melon and cantaloupe.

Muffins. Continental breakfasts are often light, focusing on breads and pastries. There is nothing wrong with baked goods; the problems start when butter or shortening is cooked in, along with all their calories. So check out our Wild Blueberry Muffin recipe (page 183). It's quick, light, and delicious, with a special trick that lets you skip the shortening. Give it a try. If you like it, let's add it to your list.

Fresh Fruit. Many people love fruit for breakfast. You cannot go wrong with cantaloupe, papayas, or mangoes. As we saw in chapter 2, the beta-carotene that gives them their bright orange color has been the focus of weight-loss studies. Combine them with bananas, grapes, or berries of all kinds. Or try oranges, or peaches.

By now you may be thinking, Wow, what a lot of carbs! Don't panic. As you will see, their calorie content is modest, their appetite-taming effect is huge, and they will give you the energy you need.

But you may want something more substantial, so read on.

Sausage and Bacon Done Healthy. If breakfast is your high-protein meal, it is easy to do sausage or bacon in a healthy, slimming way. If a typical serving (92 grams) of two pork breakfast links has 26 grams of fat, two Morningstar Farms Veggie Original Sausage Patties would deliver only 6 grams total. You could eat eight of them and still have less fat than in a pair of pork sausages (not that anyone would actually do that, one would hope). Try them or other plant-based products you may find at your regular grocery or health food store and see which ones you like.

While plant-based sausages are remarkably like meat sausages, plant-based bacon products do not aim to be an exact replica of the original. They have nonetheless become very popular and are far healthier than the meat products they replace. Try Lightlife Tempeh Smoky Bacon, Lightlife Smart Bacon, or Sweet Earth Benevolent Bacon.

Skip the poultry products. Chicken sausage and turkey bacon are processed meat products in the same cancer-causing category as pork sausage.

Breakfast Burritos. These have become a popular start to the day and a convenience food in every grocery store freezer case. They bring you the healthy fiber of beans, tofu, and vegetables. A couple of minutes in the microwave, and you have breakfast. Skip the cheesy brands.

Beans and Chickpeas. In Great Britain, baked beans are a common high-protein breakfast food. The same is true in Australia. Many American spring-breakers discover beans for breakfast in Cancún, where traditional Yucatán black beans are pureed and served with pico de gallo and chips or toast. And of course, everything in the bean group is on the power-food list.

In the Middle East, chickpeas transform into hummus, which was a breakfast tradition long before it became popular elsewhere. The healthiest hummus brands pump up the chickpeas and limit the tahini and oils. Check the labels for those lowest in fat. You can also whip up your own hummus in minutes with a food processor (see the recipe section).

Just Egg. As we saw in chapter 2, Just Egg is a convenient scrambled egg substitute that you just pour into a frying pan and scramble like an egg. It is made from mung bean protein. Other manufacturers offer similar products. Pick some up at the supermarket or health food store and see what you think.

A MOOD-BALANCING BREAKFAST

As we saw in chapter 2, some people find that starting breakfast with a plant protein (e.g., grilled tofu, grilled tempeh, veggie sausage, veggie bacon, or beans) brings a mood-balancing effect that lasts the whole day. A good order for breakfast is to start with a plant-protein food, followed by greens of any variety (e.g., broccoli, asparagus, spinach), with a carbohydrate-rich follow-up, such as cereal, oatmeal, fresh fruit, or toast. If this sounds elaborate or a bit off the beaten path, try it and see how you feel later in the day.

Scrambled Tofu. The Asian tradition of breakfast tofu has come to Europe and North America as scrambled tofu. Try a Japanese scramble for a light but delicious breakfast. You can make your own by crumbling firm tofu into a nonstick pan, with nutritional yeast, soy sauce, and, if you like, diced peppers, onions, or other veggies. As you will recall from chapter 2, Harvard researchers found that people who increase their intake of soy foods over time are slimmer than their soy-avoiding friends.

Grilled Tofu or Grilled Tempeh. These quick dishes give you a protein blast with very little fat and no cholesterol. See the recipe section for super-easy ways to prepare them.

Breakfast Vegetables. It started with onions and spinach in omelets. Then came asparagus, roasted potatoes, grilled sliced tomatoes, mushrooms, and other vegetables. Increasingly, people are including vegetables at breakfast. Don't fight it. Vegetables love you back any time of day. The key to breakfast vegetables is often the toppings. You might try "cheesy" nutritional yeast, lemon, pickles, Bragg Liquid Aminos, soy sauce, seasoned vinegar, or whatever your taste calls for.

You will find many more ideas in the recipe section.

Okay, now's the time to pick up your pen. Jot down breakfast foods that use the power foods and skip the fattening ingredients.

LIFE'S TOO SHORT

If cooking is not your thing, here is a quick rundown of breakfasts that take no time:

- Cereal (corn, wheat, oat, bran, rice, etc.) with soy milk or other plant-based milk, topped with berries or other fresh fruit. The whole-grain versions are appetite-taming, calorie-trapping foods.
- Hot cereal (oats, Cream of Wheat or grits), topped with cinnamon, black pepper, or fresh fruit.
- Frozen waffles. They are ready when the toaster pops them up. Top with syrup and berries.
- Breakfast burritos: Buy them frozen; zap when ready.
- Veggie sausage or veggie bacon: Pan frying is tastier, but microwaving is quicker.
- Just Egg: It is an eggless product that scrambles into breakfast in no time. It also comes as frozen patties to create a breakfast sandwich. Other brands are also available.
- Fresh fruit of any variety: Cantaloupe or other melon, bananas, blueberries, papayas, mangoes, oranges, apples, or whatever you fancy. All of these are power foods. If you buy a cantaloupe, cut it up as soon as you get home and keep it in a bowl in the refrigerator. A whole cantaloupe tends to be ignored, but an already-sliced one presents a handy snack.
- Toast or bagels: Favor whole-grain products to get the calorie-trapping effect.

For Liz, the research participant we met in chapter 1, having a proper breakfast was a bit of a new idea altogether. She was always at her desk well before eight a.m., so she often skipped breakfast other than a cup of coffee on the way to the office. Sometimes hunger then drove her to overdo it at lunch. During our study, she decided to get on a better track with more regular mealtimes. Some days a bowl of oatmeal did the trick, along with generous toppings. It was something she had grown up with but had let go. If she was in a hurry, she pulled an Amy's Burrito out of the freezer. It is made of beans and rice, wrapped in a tortilla, and a couple of minutes in the microwave is all it needs. She ate it in the car on the way to her office. On Saturdays, she often met friends for brunch at a restaurant. It was there she had her first taste of tofu scramble, which she quite liked.

André's mornings were different. He cooked for his wife and their two children and, after joining the research study, he just adapted their usual breakfast items. Toast was still toast, but he chose wholegrain bread and skipped the butter. He tried out a couple of different plant-based sausages and found one that everyone liked. He made home fries in a nonstick pan with diced onions and green peppers, sprinkled with paprika, and often cut up a cantaloupe or other melon. It did not feel like a diet; it was just good food.

Lunch and Dinner

Let's explore some lunch and dinner options. Think about what you eat now and how you might tweak it to power up its weight-loss potential. Let's start with a couple of everyday examples.

Power Your Pizza. Does pizza call to you? If so, the toppings make all the difference. If you were to visit any pizzeria in Rome, you would find only modest use of cheese—and none at all on some pizzas. However, in the United States, it's a different story. Chicago's Pizzeria Uno opened its doors in 1943 and featured a deep-dish pizza covered with "more cheese than people could believe," as the restaurant says, launching a yellow-asphalt orgy that would shock an

Italian pizza cook. Most pizzerias do not go that far, but they still pile on enough cheese to stop your weight-loss efforts cold.

Not only is cheese about 70 percent fat; it also contains *casomorphins,* opiates that come from dairy protein and attach to the same brain receptors that narcotics attach to, as we saw in chapter 3. Casomorphins are believed to be a driver of cheese's addictive qualities.

We can do better. Every pizzeria will gladly leave off the cheese and add extra tomato sauce with spinach, peppers, mushrooms, olives, and caramelized onions, and sometimes broccoli, eggplant, and pineapple. All the plant-based toppings have calorie-trapping fiber to carry calories away before you can absorb them. If you like a bit of spice, add diced jalapeños or a touch of sriracha sauce. As you will recall, studies suggest that the natural *capsaicin* in jalapeños and other hot peppers tames the appetite and increases metabolism.

If you are making your own pizza, nutritional yeast blends into the tomato sauce to create a remarkable cheesy flavor. It is a zero-fat, high-protein product sold at all health food stores and many regular groceries.

If convenience is the name of the game, you will find cheeseless pizzas in the freezer case. Amy's Roasted Vegetable pizza is a common brand, made with shiitake mushrooms, red onions, and fire-roasted red peppers.

Okay, that was easy. Let's try another tweak.

Top Your Spaghetti. If you normally top your spaghetti with ground-beef sauce, try a chunky marina or spicy arrabbiata sauce. Every Italian restaurant has them, and it is easy to make your own from tomatoes, fresh basil, spices, and as much or as little roasted garlic as you like. For convenience, there are many great brands on grocery shelves. Check the labels and favor those without dairy products and with as little fat as possible. And, yes, spaghetti is healthy. As we saw in chapter 2, people who include pasta in their routines tend to be slimmer than those who do not.

If a healthy pizza or spaghetti sounds like a good addition to your menu, on to your list they go. Let's try another example:

Super Chili. With a simple tweak, meat chili can transform into bean chili and become a weight-loss powerhouse. This simple switch replaces fat with appetite-taming fiber, so you fill up on far fewer calories.

For the world's fastest chili, just combine a can of black beans, a small jar of salsa, and some corn (canned or frozen), heat it on the stove, then add hot sauce to taste, lime juice, and cilantro.

In the recipe section, you will find Southwest Chili (page 214) made from black beans, tomatoes, and corn, flavored with onions, vegetable broth, and spices, with optional finely diced jalapeños for zip. Or try the Orzo Chili (page 210) with our Cornbread (page 232) or Potato Salad (page 234).

PEPPERS GO ON, WELL, EVERYTHING

The capsaicin in peppers is credited with an appetite-taming and metabolism-boosting effect. If you like a bit of spice, peppers are for more than just nachos. Let a quarter teaspoon of diced jalapeño perk up a salad. Add them to a sandwich or dip. Use them to flavor chili or spaghetti sauce. Plunk them on your veggie burger or veggie dog. Go easy—a little bit goes a long way. But you will come to appreciate the zing they bring.

Soups and Sandwiches

If your idea of lunch is a bowl of soup and a sandwich, healthful options abound. When convenience counts, a huge variety of canned, frozen, and instant soups awaits you at the store, from light miso soup mixes to split pea, lentil, bean, butternut squash, tomato, vegetable, mushroom, and noodle soups. Did you spot the power foods? Skip those with milk, meat, butter, or coconut oil (which often shows up in Thai soups). Check the recipe section for many more delicious soups.

If peanut butter and jelly are your routine, check out defatted peanut butters, called PB2 or PBfit, at the grocery store. They keep the taste and ditch the fat.

If a grilled cheese sandwich is your thing, try hummus as a sandwich filling instead. Yes, we mentioned it as a Middle Eastern breakfast food, but it's become a lunchtime staple. The chickpeas from which it is made are indeed a power food, with about 80 percent less fat than cheese. Serve it on regular bread or in a pita, adding sliced tomatoes, lettuce, cucumbers, or whatever calls to you. Or have baked falafel in a pita with a salad. Chickpeas' calorie-trapping fiber makes you feel full and satisfied.

EASY AND ELEGANT APPETIZER

If you are hosting a luncheon, here is a way to make an easy appetizer with a touch of elegance. In a food processor, a basic hummus takes about five minutes to prepare, using canned chickpeas, a touch of tahini, scallions, parsley, garlic, and black pepper (see the recipe section). The elegance comes in by offering a selection: one featuring red peppers blended in and slivered on top, one topped with pine nuts, one with beet matchsticks, and one with extra garlic. Something about offering things in colorful sets always impresses guests. If you are in a hurry, you can buy premade varieties.

Burgers. A huge array of healthy meatless versions is now readily available. Check the regular grocery store and also the health food store freezer cases. Burgers made from black beans or other plant-derived ingredients bring you appetite-taming, calorie-trapping fiber you won't find in a meat burger.

A note of caution: In recent years, the Beyond Burger and Impossible Burger have aimed to seduce meat-eaters with plant-based burgers that, while healthier than the meaty burgers they replace, have more fat than you will want, including coconut oil. Don't go there. You will find healthier brands, as you will see when you check their labels. Or you can make your own.

Hot Dogs. Plant-based hot dogs will trick even a food-dissecting eleven-year-old. Let's compare: You are at a picnic, and your host hands you a paper plate with two Oscar Mayer Original Wieners. They are made from turkey, chicken, and pork. Twenty grams of fat, and 220 calories. "What a minute," he says. "Try these instead." Now, he hands you a paper plate with two Lightlife Smart Dogs. Just 4 grams of fat and 120 calories, and they are made with soy protein, rather than meat. As you'll recall, soy products were among the foods that Harvard researchers found to be most consistently associated with weight loss. With ketchup, mustard, relish, and chopped onions, only your waistline will know the difference. Go for it.

Check out the veggie dogs at the store. Pick up a couple of different brands and see which ones you like best.

There are many, many more great lunchtime choices. Try our Oven-Baked Macaroni recipe (page 273). Nutritional yeast provides its cheesy flavor; it is entirely dairy-free. The Faux Tuna Sandwiches (page 200), Potato-Lentil Enchiladas (page 267), and Mushroom Quesadillas (page 196) are quick, light, and delicious.

A Dinner Menu

Dinnertime choices can include all those we had for lunch, but let's dress it up a bit. Let's start with a nice, hot soup. We have looked at many already as lunchtime choices. For starters, nothing beats Pasta e Fagioli (page 211) for traditional authenticity. You can see why this simple pasta and bean staple helped make southern Italy the healthy place it has been. Or try our Creamy Chipotle Butternut

Soup (page 202), or Very Fast Veggie Lentil Soup (page 204). Our Mexican Noodle Soup (page 213) draws its flavor from fire-roasted tomatoes and gentle spices.

For our salad course, how about a simple salad of butterhead lettuce, sliced cherry tomatoes, diced peppers, a sprinkle of raisins, and our Balsamic-Dijon Vinaigrette (page 303)? If you like, add chickpeas or cubes of baked tofu (available at any health food store and many regular groceries). Or try our Asian-Inspired Rice Salad (page 235) with Orange Ginger Dressing (page 305), which combines the benefits of ginger, soy, rice, and oranges; or our simple Green Bean Salad (page 233) with Balsamic-Dijon Vinaigrette. As you can see, we are putting the power ingredients to work.

In the recipe section, you will also find our Creamy Broccoli Salad (page 229), Potato Salad (page 234), Easy Quinoa and Broccoli Tabbouleh (page 216), Massaged Kale Caesar (page 217), Seaweed, Cucumber, and Chickpea Salad (page 225), and a fun Pinto Picnic Salad (page 218) made with spinach, papaya, pinto beans, and brown rice, along with lots of other choices.

DRESS UP YOUR SALAD

Salads can be healthful, of course. Let's pump up their flavor and appeal, along with their health value, with simple tweaks.

- **Go for contrasts.** Lettuce leaves have a faint bitterness. Contrast that with a sprinkle of raisins or grapes for sweetness. Lettuce leaves are also very light. Contrast this with some chickpeas for substance. Then think about adding greens, yellow cherry tomatoes, red peppers, purple beets, or blackberries. Did you spot the power ingredients?
- **Degrease it.** Leave off the cheese, bacon bits, chicken, tuna, etc.

■ **Try fancy vinegars.** If you are looking for a commercial
    salad dressing, check the vinegar section. Balsamic
    vinegar, white wine vinegar, red wine vinegar,
    champagne vinegar, aged sherry vinegar, seasoned
    rice vinegar—each one brings its own flavor without
    the fat found in oily dressings. Next to the vinegars are
    vinegar-derived glazes that are handy for vegetables.

■ **Add that extra something.** If you have not yet tried
    Bragg Liquid Aminos, it is next to the soy sauce at
    the health food store and goes great on a salad. A
    tiny dose of minced jalapeños or a sprinkle of black
    pepper makes it pop.

For a main dish, you will love the Moroccan Shepherd's Pie (page 262), the Potato-Lentil Enchiladas (page 267), the One-Pot Cauliflower Piccata Pasta (page 245), Twice-Baked Mediterranean Sweet Potatoes (page 226), Chickpea Pot Pie Stew with Herbed Polenta Dumplings (page 206), and the Speedy One-Pot Dal (page 208). The Cheesy Broccoli Casserole (page 253) is super-quick and satisfying.

For a touch of elegance when entertaining friends, try the Samosa Lettuce Cups (page 198) or the Asian-Inspired Rice Salad (page 235) with our Orange Ginger Dressing (page 305). Follow with Aloo Matar, an Indian potato, tomato, and pea curry (page 271), or Mango Dal (page 209) with Perfect Brown Rice (page 237). Or how about Baked Polenta with Mushroom Ragu (page 242) topped with Creamy Tofu Sauce (page 304), Pesto Spaghetti with Broccoli and Sun-Dried Tomatoes (page 244), Red Pepper and Artichoke Paella (page 251), or Chilled Bok Choy Soba Noodle Bowls (page 249)?

You will likely want a side of rice, corn, or a good bread, or a starchy vegetable, like a sweet potato or steamed carrots. These are all fine choices, provided you skip the butter and oil that would pack in calories.

Simplicity and Elegance

Let me share Liz's and André's experiences with planning special dinners. For Liz, it was a Super Bowl party for friends. The research study had finished. She'd maintained the healthy diet that had changed her life, and she was not about to serve chicken wings and bratwurst. Even though this was just an informal gathering around the television, she wanted to keep it healthy and also wanted to introduce her friends to some of the food tricks she had learned.

At her local grocery store, she picked up frozen MorningStar Farms Chik'n Nuggets, which taste exactly like the high-cholesterol variety, but are entirely plant-based. They heat quickly, so she planned to put them in the oven just as guests arrived. She laid out a bar of flavored dips that she found at the store: mango habanero, sweet chili, chili lime, and Hellmann's Vegan Mayo Dressing and Spread.

She asked a local pizzeria to deliver pizzas with no cheese, but with extra sauce, sautéed spinach, olives, mushrooms, and caramelized onions. When they arrived, she sprinkled on nutritional yeast for a cheesy flavor, and filled little dishes with pepperoncini for guests to add.

She also made sliders, using a quick grain and bean recipe, similar to the Weeknight Bean Burgers you'll see in the recipe section of this book (page 194). This was the one dish that actually required a little cooking. Had she been more pressed for time, she would have used frozen veggie burger patties.

She put out a pot of vegetarian baked beans that she had taken from cans, and corn on the cob that she had boiled, served with seasoned salt.

Her guests were impressed by the varied and delicious tastes, and everything disappeared quickly. After dinner, she brought out a banana split bar, where everyone could make their own, with bananas, almond milk yogurt, fresh berries, and a date caramel topping. On the way out the door, her friends agreed that this was the place to come next year, too.

Not that anyone noticed, but the power foods were clearly in evidence: The Chik'n Nuggets bring the power of soy with hot pepper toppings and their capsaicin power. The pizza skipped the fatty cheese, using all high-fiber toppings, and the sliders, baked beans, and corn on the cob followed suit. The banana split bar was as healthful as it was fun, especially with the colorful berry toppings. To Liz, healthy eating was now second nature.

André hosted a different kind of dinner. It was his parents' fiftieth wedding anniversary, and he and his siblings, nieces, and nephews wanted to create something special.

With a "Golden Anniversary" theme, he placed a bouquet of yellow roses and violets in the center of the dinner table. The first course was a yellow lentil soup with slivered red peppers on top, with red and green grapes on the side for contrast.

Next came a salad of Bibb lettuce and radicchio, topped with golden raisins and crushed walnuts, with a faintly sweet vinaigrette. An edible fresh violet blossom was atop each one.

Because his parents had married in Louisiana, the main dish was a sentimental one, jambalaya, but made with healthy ingredients— chickpeas, kidney beans, rice, green and red peppers, and onions— along with sides of red beans and rice. And dessert was sweet potato pie.

André's sister pulled out an old vinyl record by Gladys Knight & the Pips and put it on the stereo. As "The Best Thing That Ever Happened to Me" played, André hoped they had remembered right that it was the song played at their wedding reception in 1974.

As the music played, his mother spotted a tear in his father's eye. "You old softy," she said, touching his hand.

"It's André's cooking," his father said. "André's cooking is so great, it always makes me cry," he said, laughing. "No, I'm just kidding," he said. "André, bringing us all together for this lovely meal was the most beautiful thing you could have done. And all you kids are the best thing that ever happened to your mother and me."

Desserts

When it comes to dessert, often we just need to tweak a recipe to emphasize the weight-loss foods and eliminate the not so healthful ingredients. Berries bring their weight-loss power to pies, tarts, and cobblers. Cinnamon adds a delightful flavor to our Raspberry Banana Oatmeal Cookies (page 282), Quickie Cinnamon Rice Pudding (page 287), Blueberry Pear Crumble (page 280), and Quick Apple Cinnamon Skillet (page 281). Berries are featured in several of these, too, as well as in our Strawberry Banana Nice Cream (page 276), Beat the Summer Blueberry Pops (page 277), Triple-Berry No-Churn Sorbet (page 278), and Black and Blue Brownies (page 283).

And of course, the healthiest desserts—and sometimes the most satisfying—are often the simplest: Strawberries, chunks of fresh mango, and banana slices with optional sprinkled sliced almonds are tasty and leave no regrets.

Snacks

A healthy snack keeps your fires burning and prevents the exaggerated hunger that can propel overeating later. To get there, you'll want healthy complex carbohydrate for energy and fiber to tame your appetite, without a load of grease that would make you sluggish.

You already know a lot about tweaking snacks to make them more healthful. For example, if we choose baked potato chips instead of regular chips, the fat per serving drops from 10 grams to 3, and the calories drop from 160 to 120. Similarly, while regular tortilla chips have 7 grams of fat per one-ounce serving, baked tortilla chips cut that to 3 grams. This does not mean that chips are the ultimate health food, but you can see how a minor tweak from fried to baked makes a big difference. Here are more ideas:

Fresh fruit. As you know by now, bananas are great at taming the appetite with minimal calories. Apples, oranges, peaches, pears, grapes, mangoes, and all their friends in the produce aisle can jump in and help, too. Keep a good supply on hand.

Dried fruit. Raisins, apricots, dates, and other dried fruits keep well and travel well, too.

Cereal. The same cereal you may have for breakfast works any time of day.

Toast with cinnamon or jam. Skip the butter.

Rice cakes. They are filling with almost no calories. Have them plain or top them with jam or hummus.

Popcorn. Air-popped popcorn is a healthy whole grain. It is great plain or topped with cinnamon, nutritional yeast, or just a bit of salt.

Instant soups. Grocery stores stock a selection of packaged soups that come to life with hot water: miso soup, split pea, lentil, minestrone, and Asian noodle soups are all great.

Bean salad. A jar of three-bean or four-bean salad is ready when you are.

Plant-based yogurt. Soy-based yogurt packs a power ingredient and skips the disadvantages of dairy products. Check the labels and favor those lowest in fat.

Power bars. Many contain berries, whole grains, and other high-fiber ingredients, but products vary tremendously. An Oatmeal Raisin Walnut Clif bar has 6 grams of fat. Ditto for the Crunchy Peanut Butter flavor, and the same for a Chocolate Cupcake Luna Bar. But a Larabar Blueberry Muffin–flavored bar has 9 grams of fat, and the Banana Bread flavor has 10 grams. A Cranberry Almond Kind bar has 12 grams. It pays to read the labels.

LIFE'S TOO SHORT

Want to save time in food preparation? Some foods cook up almost instantly:

Frozen ready-made meals: Frozen foods make life easy.

You can microwave an Amy's enchilada dinner and have a satisfying meal in minutes. There is actually a huge range of frozen dinners, pot pies, curries, soups, stews, burgers, and burritos, along with plant-based "fish" sticks and many other products to explore in the freezer case.

Frozen ingredients: Frozen berries, vegetables, rice, etc., are next to the full meals.

Pre-chopped vegetables: While pre-cut veggies are in the freezer case, you will also find them in a salad bar.

Canned foods: You can pop open a can of refried beans, nuke some frozen rice, and crack open a salsa jar quicker than you can say, "Instant power foods!" You will find a huge range of canned lentils, beans, soups, stews, and vegetables in the supermarket. Favor low-sodium varieties.

Instant soups and noodle pots: Just add water.

Quick-cooking grains: Couscous, bulgur, and quinoa cook very quickly.

Spaghetti with sauce from a jar: Spaghetti cooks fast, and opening a jar of sauce is even faster. The variety of healthful sauces is enormous: marinara, arrabbiata, tomato-basil, mushroom, and even Parmesan-free pesto. Check the labels and skip those with meat, cheese, or substantial amounts of oil.

Quick burritos and enchiladas: Gently heat a corn or wheat tortilla and fill it with beans, salsa, lettuce, or veggies. You can do the same with pita bread.

Healthy sandwich fillings: Stores now carry plant-based versions of turkey, bologna, and other luncheon meats that you can pop between slices of bread with a bit of mustard or pickle for a healthy sandwich.

Okay, those are quick ideas. And some products need no preparation at all:

Salad bars: Many grocery stores feature hot and cold salad bars and all the makings of full meals.

Fresh fruit: Remember, apples and pears are appetite-tamers (adding them to your diet reduces your overall calorie intake). And bananas, oranges, peaches, and other fruits are similarly healthful. With fruit on hand, you will always have an appetizer, snack, and dessert ready.

Prepared foods: In a grocery's deli or refrigerator section, you will find green salads, fruit salads, hummus, vegetables, vegan yogurts, veggie sushi, and many other ready-to-eat foods.

Some foods come to you:

- Local delivery services will bring you groceries or fully prepared meals from a wide range of restaurants and grocery stores.
- MamaSezz brings you plant-based meals, ready to heat and eat. It is super convenient.
- Meal delivery kit services send you all the premeasured ingredients, ready to cook. Purple Carrot, for example, is a great way to try new, healthful, and sometimes exotic flavors. There are other services, too.

In all these categories, meals vary greatly in quality and healthfulness. Choose those that include the power foods. The best choices omit animal ingredients and oily ingredients.

Complete Nutrition

As you plan your meals, you might be wondering if you are getting all the nutrition you need. Doing so turns out to be very easy. The basic rules for good nutrition are simple:

- Include four healthy food groups—fruits, vegetables, legumes, and whole grains—each day.
- Be sure to take a vitamin B$_{12}$ supplement.

As you plan your meals, think about these four healthful food groups. You will want to include them all in your routine.

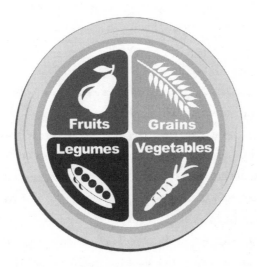

Vegetables. Vegetables provide vitamins and minerals, as you know. They also have a surprising amount of protein, complex carbohydrate, and fiber. It pays to be generous with your vegetable servings. Why not have two or three vegetables at a meal? Orange vegetables, such as carrots or sweet potatoes, go great with green vegetables, such as broccoli, Swiss chard, spinach, or asparagus.

Grains. Grains bring you healthy complex carbohydrate, protein, and fiber. While we think of grains as a breakfast food—cereals, oatmeal, pancakes—grains are a great addition to all meals. They are the main staple of the slimmest populations on the planet. You are already familiar with rice, wheat, corn, oats, etc. If you are feeling adventurous, try quinoa, millet, barley, bulgur, amaranth, etc.

Beans and other legumes. Beans, peas, and lentils are rich in
   protein, minerals, and appetite-taming fiber. Bean products,
   such as tofu or tempeh, have health benefits of their own.
Fruit. Fruit is a great source of vitamins and fiber and makes a
   great dessert or snack, packed with weight-loss power.

Vitamin B$_{12}$ is used by your body to form red blood cells and also
for healthy nerve function. It is a curious vitamin because it is not
made by plants or animals. It is made by bacteria. Scientists believe
that, long ago, we humans got traces of vitamin B$_{12}$ from bacteria in
the soil, on our hands, in our mouths, and so on. If that was ever
true, modern hygiene has eliminated these sources.

Vitamin B$_{12}$ is added to many breakfast cereals, soy milk, and
other foods, but you should not count on these as consistent sources.
Animal products contain B$_{12}$ because their gut bacteria make it. Ours
do, too, but it appears that the B$_{12}$ in our intestines is formed too far
along to be readily absorbed.

The safest thing is to take a B$_{12}$ supplement. Do not neglect this.
The US government already recommends one for adults over fifty,
and that is good advice for everyone. The Recommended Dietary
Allowance is tiny—just 2.4 micrograms per day. B$_{12}$ is in all daily
multivitamins, as well as in supplements of B$_{12}$ alone, which are
sold in all drugstores, grocery stores, and health food stores. Supplements of 100 to 200 micrograms are fine for daily use. Larger
supplements—1,000 micrograms or greater—can be used every
other day (or at whatever frequency your doctor recommends if it is
part of a medical regimen).

The reason for caution about higher doses, apart from the fact
that it is best not to overdo it on any vitamins, is that some evidence
has suggested that overdosing on vitamins B$_6$ and B$_{12}$ may be associated with higher risk of fractures.[1] We need to stay tuned for clearer
evidence, but while scientists sort it out, it is a good idea to get the
vitamins you need and avoid excesses.

Let's talk about the subjects of common nutrition questions: protein, calcium, and iron.

Protein. You need protein to repair body tissues and to build certain hormones and enzymes. Some people think of meat or eggs as providing protein, vegetables as providing vitamins, and starchy foods as providing calories. However, all of these foods have protein. In fact, the protein in grains, beans, vegetables, and fruits turns out to be better for you than the protein in meat or eggs—or, for that matter, in power bars or protein shakes.

As we saw in chapter 3, Harvard's Nurses' Health Study and Health Professionals Follow-Up Study found that replacing animal-derived protein with plant protein was associated with reduced mortality.[2] Specifically, people favoring plant sources of protein tended to be healthy, while those getting their protein from red meat, fish, poultry, dairy products, or eggs were more likely to have their lives shortened by heart problems and other diseases. Other studies have shown the same thing.[3]

There is no need for animal protein, and you are far better off without it. A diet drawn from any normal variety of plant foods gives you all the protein you need. That is true at all stages of life and regardless of whether you are sedentary or an elite athlete.

Calcium. Many of us grew up with the idea that milk is a good source of calcium. However, calcium is an element found in the earth; it is not made by cows. Plants take it up through their roots, and it ends up in their leaves. When we eat broccoli, collard greens, brussels sprouts, kale, or other plants, we use that calcium for shoring up our bones and other functions.

The only reason milk contains calcium is because cows eat plants, and the percentage you absorb from milk is lower than from most greens. For example, you absorb 64 percent of the calcium from brussels sprouts but only 32 percent from milk.

There are a couple of exceptions, however: Unlike other vegetables, spinach and chard contain calcium that is not very absorbable, though they are healthful in other respects. You'll also find calcium in beans and other legumes, soy milk, tofu, and many other foods.

The bigger reason to choose greens rather than milk is that greens give you nutrition you need—lots of fiber, beta-carotene, and vitamins. Milk's main nutrients are sugar, fat, and animal protein, along with cholesterol and estradiol—all things you can do without. And it never has the fiber you need. As you know by now, milk-drinking increases the risk of prostate and breast cancer; vegetables and beans reduce these risks.

Iron. Your red blood cells use iron to build hemoglobin, which carries oxygen to your brain and all the rest of you. Like calcium, iron is a natural element in the earth, and plants absorb it through their roots. Again, green vegetables are a rich source (and here, spinach and chard count as good sources, too), as are beans.

While many of us grew up with the idea of getting iron from meat or liver, the only reason these products have iron is that animals eat iron-containing plants.

The iron in plants, called *non-heme* iron, is the form your body was designed for, so to speak. If you are low in iron, your body absorbs more of it. If you have a lot of iron on board already, your body automatically adjusts to absorb less of it. That is great, because your body needs to be able to regulate how much iron it takes in. In large amounts, iron becomes toxic. It sparks the production of compounds called free radicals that circulate in the blood, damaging the blood vessels, heart, brain, skin, and all the rest of you.

Meat has a form of iron called *heme* iron that your body is unable to regulate. Even if you have plenty of iron on board already, meat-based iron just waltzes right into your bloodstream, ready to cause problems. By the way, dairy products interfere with iron absorption. A glass of milk with a meal cuts iron absorption in half.

If you are low in iron for any reason, your doctor will need to investigate why. If the problem is that you are missing out on greens and beans, it is easy to fix. If you are losing iron from excessive menstrual flow, a low-fat plant-based diet often helps, surprisingly enough, making periods more regular, less protracted, and less painful. Your doctor will also check to see if you are losing blood for some other reason. Only rarely is an iron supplement necessary.

NUTRITION FOR CHILDREN

Children are at ever-increasing risk for weight problems, thanks to the marketing of cheese, meat, and unhealthy snack foods. Those who are lucky enough to grow up on plant-based diets have a huge health advantage. They are more likely to stay healthy and to avoid excessive weight gain. For children who have developed weight problems, a low-fat, plant-based diet helps enormously. Rather than focus on the child, though, the entire family should adopt the same healthful diet.

The nutrition rules for children are more or less the same as for adults: Build your nutrition from the four healthy food groups and take a B_{12} supplement, which could be any typical children's multivitamin.

Remember, our goal with this chapter has been to become familiar with meals that incorporate the power foods and eliminate unhealthful ingredients. If you have not yet picked up your pen and paper, now is a perfect time to jot down the foods that might work for you and to test them out. As you involve your family or friends in the process, you'll get even more ideas and will get them excited about the power of food for health, too.

In the next chapter, we'll go out on the town and see what foods are in store for us.

CHAPTER 6

Eating on the Go

Modern life often means eating at restaurants, on airplanes, in the car, at our desks, or relying on food-delivery services. Luckily, there is an abundance of healthful foods available for all of these situations. In this chapter, we will find them. With a few simple tips, you will learn how to choose the best restaurants. We will also look at travel and vacations. There is no need to miss a beat in your weight loss at holiday times or on a family getaway. A little planning makes it easy.

Restaurants

Tip number one in choosing a good restaurant is to "think international." Many cultures incorporate healthful weight-loss ingredients into their traditional foods, and restaurateurs will gladly bring them to your table.

Francesca, a research participant we met in chapter 1, introduced us to her favorite Italian restaurant. The occasion was a reunion of the research group after the study's conclusion. The chef, Matteo, welcomed the guests, and once everyone had arrived and was seated, Francesca walked us through her menu favorites.

"You will like the bruschetta," she said, carefully accentuating the "k" sound in case anyone wanted to pronounce it "brushetta." "It's simple—just toasted bread with tomatoes and fresh basil and some garlic. But to keep it authentic, you need to start with a good bread. Matteo, what kind of bread do you use?"

"It's a baguette from the French bakery," he replied. "But for you, I left off the oil."

"For an Italian meal, you use French bread?" Francesca asked. "Anyway," she continued, "there's also a little garlic, and you'll like it."

The truth, of course, is that bruschetta, like many "traditional" foods, is actually a hybrid. French bread works fine. The tomatoes are a New World import. Basil originated in India.

Francesca pointed out the healthy salads and, of course, delicious soups: minestrone, lentil, or pasta e fagioli. She pointed out the endless pasta varieties and sauces. "Matteo will make you an arrabbiata sauce, marina sauce, or even a pesto without cheese." She asked the chef what vegetables were on hand, and he replied that he had grilled asparagus, broccolini, and spinach.

Everyone's mouths were watering. "Sometimes you have to convince the chef not to soak everything in olive oil," Francesca said. "They *love* their olive oil." She winked at Matteo. "But here it's no problem."

She was right. As Francesca said, you can ask the chef to skip the oil and to serve sauces on the side, so you can add the amount you want.

"If you want a pizza," she continued, "you can leave off the cheese, or you can go half and half, if you are sharing." Top with spinach, mushrooms, sun-dried tomatoes, eggplant, sautéed onions, bell peppers, jalapeños, or pepperoncini flakes.

Italian restaurants do indeed have lots of great options. And so do many other cuisines. Let's leave our friends to their meal and check out our other restaurant choices.

Mexican restaurants feature bean burritos, veggie fajitas, spinach enchiladas, and beans and rice, and are a perfect opportunity to show off your knowledge of hot peppers and their capsaicin-fueled weight-loss potential. Skip the cheese. As we have seen, most good Mexican restaurants do not put lard in beans, but a few still do. It pays to ask.

In my childhood home of Fargo, North Dakota, the Mexican Village restaurant serves a jalapeño burrito made of refried beans and a not-quite-life-threatening quantity of jalapeños wrapped in a tortilla and covered with a delicious gravy. If you leave off the cheese sprinkles, it is entirely plant-based. For less adventurous diners, it is okay to leave off the jalapeños.

Other Latin American restaurants reflect their own traditions. Cuban restaurants, for example, always feature traditional black beans, along with plantains and salads, while Argentinean restaurant menus are more meat-heavy.

Japanese cuisine is a gold mine of healthful choices that are typically prepared without added oils. Start with edamame—the steamed baby soy pods—and add a bowl of miso soup. It is sometimes prepared with fish flavoring and sometimes not, so you will want to ask. Follow with a green salad or, for extra points, a seaweed salad. As you will recall, vegetables from the sea provide iodine, the essential ingredient for thyroid hormone, which controls your metabolism. Or have a light cucumber or spinach salad.

Next up, let's see what the sushi chef has in mind. A cucumber roll, an asparagus roll, a sweet potato roll, or other veggie rolls are light and delicious. And yes, their nori wrappers are iodine-rich, too, and the tangy pickled ginger condiment has weight-loss properties of its own, as we saw in chapter 2.

Chinese restaurants have delicious soups as starters, followed by a range of rice dishes, of course. Rice is one of the reasons that people in Japan and other Asian countries are among the healthiest, longest-lived people on the planet. There are also many noodle dishes, which are similarly healthful. They feature familiar vegetables like broccoli, spinach, and green beans, as well as some that are new to many Westerners, and delicately prepared tofu.

CHINESE VEGETABLES

Many Chinese restaurants have special menus for their Chinese customers featuring vegetables that are not listed on the regular menu. These are not side dishes. They are front and center, steamed or sautéed with garlic, and eaten along with rice, tofu, and other dishes. Let's stop in at Good Friends restaurant In Brighton, England, where the staff will help us get to know some delicious vegetables, along with their Cantonese names:

Bok choy (白菜) means "white vegetable." You know this one already.

Tong choy (冬菜) means "hollow vegetable" and is sometimes called morning glory or water spinach. With its thin stalks and soft leaves, it is a great choice for people who are new to Chinese vegetables.

Si yong choy (西洋菜) means "vegetable from the west ocean" and is actually watercress. It is sautéed or served in soups.

Choy sum (菜心) means "vegetable heart." It is typically boiled and served with a light sauce.

Gai-lan (芥蘭) means "mustard orchid" and is also called Chinese broccoli. It is similar to broccoli rabe, but sweeter.

Dau myoo (豆苗) are the shoots that come from the plants that produce mange-tout pea pods.

Next time you visit a Chinese restaurant, ask about these items. Your server can tell you which vegetables are in season. Favor smaller varieties (e.g., baby bok choi); you will find they are especially tender and delicious.

Hot pot restaurants have the most delicious, most healthful, and hands-down most fun food in many cities, even if it is also the least known. Diners gather around a table outfitted with cauldrons of boiling broth, adding ingredients that cook quickly, ready to be scooped out, seasoned, and consumed with delight. It is a party as much as a meal.

Hot pot's roots are in China, beginning as bronze pots perched on tripods over small stoves. Time brought the custom to Taiwan, Japan, Thailand, the Philippines, and finally the United States.

This is not the same as the hot stone bowls—sometimes called "hot pots"—of rice and veggies served in many Asian restaurants. Delicious as they are as rice caramelizes along the bottom of the burning-hot bowl, they are entirely different from what is served in a hot pot restaurant. Here, you'll do the cooking.

At many hot pot restaurants, diners pay an all-you-can-eat price for absurdly generous stacks of raw steak, pork belly, beef tongue, tripe, beef artery, duck blood, and various vegetable afterthoughts to send into the boiling broth. So can this tradition really be done without all that meat? The answer is, of course! Hot pot restaurants are way ahead of you, with a smorgasbord of main dishes, savory and sweet sauces, and desserts, all animal-free.

Start with a healthy soup base: miso, mushroom, tomato, or pickled sour broth. Add delicate bean curd sticks, frozen tofu, firm tofu, or fried tofu, all in bite-sized pieces, and some mushrooms— king, enoki, or black mushrooms.

Lotus root, taro root, and winter melon add substance and subtle flavors of their own. But don't miss the sweet potatoes and pumpkins sliced so razor-thin they will vanish if not scooped promptly from the broth.

Next, add the superb greens. Baby bok choy comes into its own in mushroom broth. And don't miss tong ho, also called crown daisy or chrysanthemum garland, which quickly cooks to perfection. You will also find napa cabbage, broccoli, and bean seedlings. Enjoy these with rice or noodles.

What turns these elements into a masterpiece is your personal sauce, created at the seasoning bar. A simple combination of soy sauce, minced garlic, sesame seeds, cilantro, scallions, and a few crumbled peanuts gets the job done, and you will also find sriracha sauce, shredded radish, barbecue sauce, and many other tastes.

Dinner is followed by desserts that are soft-spoken, compared with ice cream and cake. A Washington, DC–area hot pot restaurant features shaved ice with fruity flavors and its signature black sugar ice pudding. Looking like a floating ice cube with a hint of tan underneath, it is actually a transparent bit of magic made from ground konjac, a distinctive flower whose underground tuber makes a plant version of gelatin. A spoonful of brown sugar hides underneath and makes it perfect.

Hot pot is an adventure. Along the way, it gives us a cornucopia of fiber-rich vegetables, along with the benefits of rice and soy products, and makes it easy to skip the fattening ingredients. Invite friends.

Google "hot pot" and the name of the city you are in to see if there is one nearby.

Korean, Thai, and Vietnamese restaurants have many healthful dishes featuring noodles, rice, vegetables, and tofu with delicate sauces, as well as salads and soups.

Indian restaurants start with simple treasures—lentils, chickpeas, potatoes, spinach, cauliflower, and other healthful foods—and build them into masterpieces, accompanied by soups, rice, and various breads. Ask for dairy-free and reduced-oil portions, since many Indian cooks indulge in dairy products and oils, which contribute to health problems.

Middle Eastern fare is now familiar, featuring falafel, hummus, tabouleh, and other foods based on simple, plant-based ingredients.

Ethiopian restaurants flourish in Washington, DC, Los Angeles, New York, and many other cities. You can take advantage of the fact that many Ethiopians avoid animal products for religious reasons on Wednesdays and Fridays, throughout Lent, and on other days as well, so Ethiopian restaurants have a huge array of traditional healthy foods on the menu. The presentation is as delightful as the food itself. A huge platter is topped with injera, a soft bread, and various foods are placed on top: lentils, split peas, potatoes, cabbage, and green beans. You will notice that hot peppers and their capsaicin have arrived in Ethiopia, too. Tear off a piece of injera, use it to scoop up whichever food calls to you, and pop it into your mouth.

Family-style restaurants and diners may surprise you. Take a lesson from Denny's. The restaurant chain started out in 1953 in California as Danny's Donuts. Later on, Danny's became Denny's, and the doughnut shop transformed into a twenty-four-hour restaurant. So if Denny's can change its stripes, it can also change what it puts on your table. No, it's not all bacon, eggs, and burgers. Try this at any family restaurant or diner, and you will see what I mean.

At breakfast, you can go basic with oatmeal, grits, or Cream of Wheat topped with blueberries, bananas, or whatever is on offer. Or you can order the healthiest meal imaginable: Ask your server for asparagus or spinach, along with grilled mushrooms, tomatoes, and whole-grain toast. Yes, they keep them in stock for making omelets, and you're just skipping the egg. Many places now serve cholesterol-free veggie sausages, like the ones from MorningStar Farms. For lunch or dinner, they offer veggie burgers, stir-fries, spaghetti with tomato sauce, and various salads and side vegetables.

Steak houses may seem like the last place one would come for a healthy meal. But their menus invariably feature a selection of healthful side dishes, such as grilled asparagus, spinach, sweet potato puree, corn on the cob, and other items that can be combined to make a vegetable plate. Menus also often include entrée-sized salads.

Soul food. The NuVegan Café in Washington, DC, has served Beyoncé, Jay-Z, many other celebrities, and a long line of everyday folks who love their sweet kale salads, collard greens, pancakes, waffles, grits, biscuits, cinnamon rolls, chick'n drummies, lasagna, vegan crab cakes, mac and vegan cheese, and a seemingly endless menu of traditional soul food and other items. There are actually many fully plant-based soul food restaurants in cities across the United States. A quick Google search will show you.

Vegan restaurants featuring foods drawn from many different traditions are now very common. You can find them in your local area by searching online. But keep in mind that vegan dishes of various kinds are available at most restaurants nowadays, as we have seen in the examples above.

DEGREASING YOUR MEAL

While restaurateurs have come to understand the desire for meatless meals, most are a bit slow to understand the value of limiting oil, as Francesca reminded us. Oil is healthier than animal fats, but when it comes to calories it is as fattening as butter or chicken fat. Here are some tips for minimizing oils at restaurants:

- Top salads with vinegar instead of oily dressings. Vinegars have gotten fancier over the years; see what they have on hand. Or use a spritz or two of juice from a lemon wedge.
- Ask that dressings and sauces be served on the side, so you can use the amount you want.
- Order vegetables steamed instead of sautéed. Potatoes can be baked, roasted, steamed, or boiled.
- Ask the server if the kitchen can minimize the use of oil in your meal.

Extra Tips for Restaurants

By choosing the right kind of restaurant, you are much more likely to have a healthy meal and a great experience. Here are a few more tips:

Go beyond the menu. Restaurants often have food items that never make it to the menu, so it is good to ask. It is surprising to find how many restaurants will readily prepare oatmeal at breakfast, a veggie burger at lunch, or spaghetti with tomato sauce at dinner, even if these items are not on the menu.

Check cooking methods. Items that are baked, roasted, broiled, grilled, poached, steamed, or stir-fried will typically use less oil than those that are deep-fried.

Order a vegetable plate. While it might sound modest, you will come to appreciate the healthfulness and flavor of a vegetable plate. Chefs are glad to provide potatoes, beans, chickpeas, broccoli, asparagus, sweet potatoes, spinach, corn on the cob, carrots, pasta salad, and other healthful items. Ask for the items you'd like.

Keep your momentum going. At restaurants, it can be tempting to throw caution to the wind "just this once" and indulge in something you know you will regret later. There is a lot to be said for sticking to your resolve to eat healthfully.

Get a box. Restaurant portions continue to grow, and servers are glad to provide to-go boxes. By all means use them.

Tip generously. The second time you dine at a restaurant, you will be glad you tipped well the first time. Your server and the kitchen crew will be eager to help with any special requests.

Fast Food

Fast-food outlets sell a lot of things that carry our health in the wrong direction. In the United States, that is partly the government's fault.

Odd as it may sound, US law requires that the government promote American agricultural products,[1] and the US Department of Agriculture has been especially eager to contract with major fast-food chains to increase the amount of cheese they sell. A surprising number of menu items have been introduced in this way: Wendy's Cheddar Lover's Bacon Cheeseburger, Subway's Chicken Cordon Bleu and Honey Pepper Melt, Pizza Hut's Ultimate Cheese Pizza (with an entire pound of cheese on a single serving), and various items at Burger King, Taco Bell, and elsewhere. No, they are not designed for health. They are designed to boost industry income. Nowadays, instead of cheese being an option on a sandwich, it comes routinely, and diners have to specifically ask if they want to avoid it.

Nonetheless, it is indeed possible to eat healthfully at fast-food restaurants. Here are several examples.

Subway and **Quiznos** make healthy eating easy. Pick out your bread, ask for all the veggie toppings: lettuce, fresh spinach, tomato, cucumbers, olives, hot peppers, and red wine vinegar. Skip the oil.

Taco Bell offers a bean burrito, which, if you hold the cheese, makes a reasonably healthful meal. Add jalapeños if you like. The seven-layer burrito is a fancier variation on the theme (skip the cheese and sour cream). Add a serving of rice.

Chipotle makes burritos and bowls with black or pinto beans, rice, veggies, various toppings, and a full range of salsas.

Domino's will gladly prepare a healthy pizza. Start with the crunchy thin crust, and top it with robust tomato sauce, Italian dipping sauce, hot buffalo sauce, garlic dipping sauce, or barbecue sauce, and add whatever toppings call to you: spinach, mushrooms, jalapeños, green peppers, roasted red peppers, banana peppers, diced tomatoes, onions, black olives, or pineapple. You can also get spaghetti marinara with all the vegetable toppings, or a Mediterranean veggie sandwich (hold the cheese).

KFC offers baked beans, corn on the cob, sweet kernel corn, green beans, side salads, and applesauce.

Wendy's has baked potatoes, side salads, and apple bites. It also has more elaborate salads, which can be made healthier by omitting cheese, bacon, chicken, and so on.

Other fast-food restaurants have been less accommodating.

Burger King offers a side salad that can be ordered without cheese, and applesauce. Regrettably, BK's veggie burger is the Impossible Burger, a product that is packed with coconut oil, aiming to seduce meat-eaters. As you will recall, coconut oil is very high in saturated ("bad") fat, along with plenty of calories, and is best avoided completely. You can, of course, order a burger or Whopper with no patty, cheese, or mayo—basically bread and condiments.

McDonald's has a fruit and maple oatmeal that can be ordered without cream. You'll also find apple slices. Like Burger King, your sandwich option is a burger with no patty, but with pickles, lettuce, onion, and the like.

FAST FOOD AT THE GROCERY STORE!

Many grocery stores have extensive hot and cold salad bars that can provide a lightning-fast meal. Check your watch as you park your car. Then cruise through the salad items—lettuce, tomatoes, chickpeas, three-bean salad—and all the soups and hot items, and head for the checkout. You will have a remarkably healthy meal in hand and be back in your car in no time!

Travel and Vacations

Travel and vacations are times when many people gain weight that never quite comes off. That does not have to happen. With a little planning, travel's challenges can be dealt with.

Of course, travel means restaurants, and you are already an expert there. And here are more tips to help no matter where you travel.

In the Car. If you have a long drive ahead of you, you might want to keep some snacks on hand:

- Bananas are nature's power bar. They are healthy, filling, easily digestible, and, as we have seen, great for weight control. Power bars themselves are handy, but check the labels to avoid the fattier brands, as we saw in chapter 5.
- Apples, pears, oranges, grapes, fruit cups, and applesauce are also great in the car. Baby carrots give you a dose of beta-carotene wherever you are.
- Raisins and other dried fruits are handy, tasty, and rich in healthy fiber.
- Rice cakes are filling and easy to handle. Bring along some bean dip, if you like.
- Small cartons of soy milk, almond milk, or fresh juice are handy, too.

On the Plane. Here are some ideas that help during air travel:

- On international flights, you can get a special meal provided you request it at least forty-eight hours in advance. The vegan meal is the healthiest option.
- On shorter flights, in-flight options are often limited, so you might want to pack any of the snack items mentioned above—just don't put a banana at the bottom of your suitcase. Or how about a sandwich with hummus or a PB and J, or a healthy sub?
- At larger airports, you will find a range of restaurants, where all the above tips apply.

At the Hotel. When it comes to healthy eating, there are many ways to make a hotel a bit more like home:

- Most medium-priced hotels in the United States have in-room refrigerators. If yours does not, request one. Many hotels have a supply of mini refrigerators for people who need to store insulin. Many hotels also have microwave ovens.
- Hotels designed for longer stays have full kitchenettes. A quick trip to the local grocery will have you set.
- Hotel restaurants often have limited menus, and the same is true for room service. But if you don't see what you want, by all means ask.
- Have it delivered. Ask the front desk for a list of restaurants that deliver, and your order of Szechuan tofu and broccoli in garlic sauce will be at your door in minutes, along with a fortune cookie.

If you are at a convention or other work-related meeting, it pays to plan ahead. I recently attended a medical meeting that took place at a steak house, a regrettably common occurrence. I called the venue ahead of time and asked if they had a vegetable plate. The manager said, "Sure. And you are the third call I've had about that today." Sure enough, when the meeting time came, many attendees had requested healthy meals.

At a catered conference, caterers are used to dealing with special requests of all kinds. Vegan meals are among the most common requests. You might also want to bring along some fresh fruit or a sandwich for snack time.

Dining at restaurants and during travel is never as predictable as eating in your own home, and curveballs are to be expected. It pays to think ahead, and to have a sense of humor when things do not go quite right. With these tricks, you'll be able to enjoy the adventure.

CHAPTER 7

Go for the Max

In chapter 5, I mentioned an exciting way to bring extra power to your efforts to improve your eating habits. It is a simple immersion in which you follow for twenty-one days what is as close to a perfect diet as possible. It not only shows you the power of healthy eating; it also gives your tastes and preferences a healthy reboot. For many people, it is a life-changing experience. We will break the process into two steps:

Step One: Explore Your Possibilities. This step lasts one week. Over the next seven days, think about meals that use the power foods as much as possible, include no animal products, and keep oils very low. As you can see, the focus on plant-based foods increases your intake of appetite-taming fiber, and, if there are no animal products or added oils in your diet, you will greatly reduce fat and all the dense calories it holds.

For most of us, it is a new idea to have no meat, dairy products, or eggs for even a day, let alone twenty-one days. But these products slow down your weight-loss efforts and have other health consequences you do not want. It pays to set them aside. As you will see, this is a powerful and engaging exercise.

As I mentioned in chapter 5, it is a good idea to write down your ideas for breakfast, lunch, dinner, and snacks, and you may have started your list already. Think about foods you can eat at home, at restaurants, or wherever you are likely to be. In the preceding chapters, we have seen lots of ideas for healthy meals, including many that require little or no cooking, and many great choices at restaurants, too. For any that are new to you, test them out this week.

Soon, you will have an impressive list of foods that bring weight-loss power and exclude the ingredients that get in the way. You will have explored them at the store and know which ones you like.

Step Two: A Three-Week Test-Drive. Now that you have picked out your favorites from the foods that propel weight loss, let's put them to work in a short test. For the next twenty-one days, have plenty of vegetables, fruits, whole grains, beans, and all the meals they turn into, and skip animal-derived products and oily foods altogether. At this point, this should actually be easy. After all, you can do anything for three weeks, and you already have your list. You have probably stocked up on many of these foods, too.

Keep in mind, this is just a short test. You are not making a plan for the rest of your life. For three weeks, do this 100 percent, so you can really see its power.

At the end of three weeks, two things will have happened. First, you will have lost weight. Whether it is a little or a lot, you will notice that the weight loss came without hunger and without adding any exercise. It was essentially automatic. You may also have noticed health changes: better energy, sounder sleep, better digestion, and, if you have diabetes, better blood sugar values. If you like what is happening, let's keep going. Your benefits will continue to grow, and you will find more and more food items to explore.

The 3-Gram Trick

To maximize your results, use the 3-Gram Trick. In chapter 3, I mentioned how fats and oils are packed with calories. Fats also cause

MY FOOD IDEAS

Breakfast

Old-fashioned oatmeal with blueberries
French toast with cinnamon, sliced banana, and maple syrup
Cornflakes with soy milk and raspberries
Veggie sausage
Breakfast burrito
Half cantaloupe
Toast with blackberry jam

Lunch

Garden salad with red wine vinegar
Veggie chili
Split pea or tomato soup with crackers
Bean burrito with salsa and diced jalapeños
Hummus sandwich with lettuce and tomato
PB&J
At Subway: veggie sub

Dinner

Minestrone, lentil, or butternut squash soup
Pizza with mushrooms, spinach, and green peppers
Moroccan Shepherd's Pie (page 262)
Potato-Lentil Enchiladas (page 267)

At Italian restaurant: angel hair pasta with arrabbiata sauce and grilled
spinach; or linguine with artichoke hearts and seared oyster mushrooms

At sushi bar: miso soup, edamame, green salad, cucumber roll, and sweet
    potato roll
Steamed broccoli, spinach, or kale

Snacks

Bananas, apples, oranges
Instant noodle soup
Three-bean salad
Cereal with soy milk or almond milk

other problems—interfering with blood sugar control and aggravating hormone-related conditions (e.g., menstrual pain).

In our research studies, we give our participants a specific target. The idea is to have no more than 3 grams of fat per serving of food and no more than about 30 grams of fat per day. That target allows enough fat for the body's needs, but avoids the excess. Here's what this means in practice:

- Nearly all fruits, vegetables, beans, and whole grains are fine—well under 3 grams of fat per serving. Have as much of these foods as you want. The exceptions are avocados and coconuts, both of which are high in fat. For now, skip them.
- Nuts, seeds, and products made from them (e.g., peanut butter, tahini) are high in fat. Their fat is "good" (unsaturated) fat, but *all* fats still harbor 9 calories in every gram and will get in the way of efforts to lose weight. Do not rule them out forever, but during your three-week test-drive, it pays to set them aside so your taste buds can learn lower-fat preferences.
- For packaged foods, check the label for total fat content. If a serving has 3 grams of fat or less, it's fine.

The 3-Gram Trick is a powerful way to accelerate weight loss. At the same time, it can be challenging if packaged foods are a big part of your purchases; manufacturers love to add fatty ingredients to products of all kinds. But if you check food labels, you will find what you want.

Note that this does not mean you should have less than 3 grams of fat *per meal*. It means 3 grams for each of the foods that go into a meal. It is a somewhat arbitrary figure, but it gets you where you need to be.

If, at any point, your weight-loss efforts seem to stall, jot down the foods you have been eating over the preceding day or two and look for foods that break the rule. You will find them: peanut butter,

Nutrition Facts

About 30 servings per container

Serving size ½ cup dry (40g)

Amount per serving

Calories   **150**

	% Daily Value
Total Fat 3g	4%
Saturated Fat 0.5g	3%
Trans Fat 0g	
Polyunsaturated fat 1g	
Monounsaturated fat 1g	
Cholesterol 0mg	0%
Sodium 0mg	0%
Total Carbohydrate 27g	10%
Dietary Fiber 4g	13%
Soluble Fiber 2g	
Total Sugars 1g	11%
Includes 0g Added Sugars	0%
Protein 5g	

oily foods, avocados, or maybe that "just this once" slice of gooey cheese pizza. The idea is not to say "never" to these foods—that's up to you—but to set them aside for now.

Extra Benefits

As your food adventure continues, shedding unwanted weight is just the beginning. From the moment you let the power foods into your life and kick unhealthful foods to the curb, your body will begin to transform.

Ending Heartburn. If you have heartburn (gastroesophageal reflux, or GERD), it will likely go away.

Better Sleep. If you have sleep apnea, it is likely to improve as your weight falls.

Lower Cholesterol. If your cholesterol is higher than it should be, it will very likely start to drop decisively. That is because if you are avoiding animal products and added oils, your diet has essentially no cholesterol in it and very little saturated fat, which is a major driver of cholesterol production in your body. Give it several weeks to see the full effect.

A low cholesterol protects your heart, as you already know. It also protects your brain. Researchers at Kaiser Permanente checked cholesterol levels on 9,844 people in their early forties. Three decades later, it was clear that those who'd had low cholesterol levels in midlife were significantly less likely to end up with dementia.[1]

In addition, if you no longer need medications for your cholesterol, you can avoid the weight gain that comes from statin drugs (see chapter 4). By the way, this does not mean that cholesterol-lowering drugs have no role in medical practice. For some people they are potentially lifesaving. However, most people on statins would not need them if they avoided foods that contain saturated fat and cholesterol.

Improving or Reversing Diabetes. If you have type 2 diabetes, a low-fat, plant-based diet is the regimen of choice. In 2006, our research, funded by the National Institutes of Health, showed that this sort of diet controls blood sugar three times more effectively than the typical portion-controlled diet prescribed at many clinics.[2] In fact, the diet is so powerful that individuals very often need to reduce or even discontinue their medication to prevent their blood sugars from running *too low*. In other words, the diet is restoring your body's normal blood sugar control, and your medications are now too strong for you and need to be cut back. Be sure to speak with your personal physician about this and follow your doctor's recommendations. Everyone's needs are different.

The same diet changes can also be used for type 1 diabetes, allowing many people to increase their carbohydrate intake and reduce their insulin doses. Be sure to talk with your doctor along the way to modify your medication regimen as needed.

Improved Blood Pressure. If your blood pressure is up, the diet improvements you are making are likely to bring it down. This is partly because of a specific effect of vegetables and fruits on blood pressure, often attributed to their potassium content. However, by avoiding animal products and other fatty foods, the blood becomes less *viscous*—that is, less thick—so it circulates more easily and blood pressure gradually falls. Also, your continuing weight loss will bring your blood pressure down further.

If you are taking blood pressure medications, you will want to be aware of the blood pressure–lowering effect of a plant-based diet. If you continue taking your current blood pressure medications while you are improving your diet, one day you may end up lightheaded, with a blood pressure that is too low. The answer is not to adjust your medications on your own. Rather, be sure your doctor monitors your blood pressure and adjusts your doses when necessary. That is an important rule for any condition: Continue seeing your personal physician, taking your medications, and caring for your health appropriately. Change your medications in consultation with your personal physician if and when the time is right.

Better Mood. As your diet improves, you may also find that your mood improves, too. Several studies have shown that as people eject animal products from their routines and bring in plant-based foods in a big way, depression and anxiety tend to subside.[3]

This is wonderful for people who have experienced weight gain caused by antidepressants. Weight gain is common with paroxetine (Paxil), citalopram (Celexa), amitriptyline (Elavil), and nortriptyline (Pamelor), and less so with fluoxetine (Prozac) or sertraline (Zoloft). If a diet change can reduce the need for medications, so much the better.

Explore New Resources

Explore websites, books, videos, and social media pages that discuss healthful eating, particularly plant-based eating. There is now a huge selection. Dustin Harder and Lindsay S. Nixon, who are the geniuses behind the recipes in this book, have books, websites, and great programs of their own.

At the Physicians Committee, our *Exam Room* podcast, hosted by Chuck Carroll, brings you a steady stream of information and support. You can join in the chat and have your questions answered. Our Food for Life classes have a large and growing curriculum and are a great resource. You will see a huge list of in-person and online classes at PCRM.org. Just search for "Food for Life." We also launched One Healthy World as a way to bring nutrition information to people worldwide. The program is in English, Spanish, and French, with additional information in Mandarin and for people in the Indian subcontinent. For medical professionals, our annual International Conference on Nutrition in Medicine and our other continuing medical education courses are very popular.

My own books and videos cover a wide variety of health issues, including weight loss, diabetes, brain health, tackling chronic pain, and dealing with hormonal issues. Have a look.

For people who need medical or dietetic care, we launched the Barnard Medical Center, a nonprofit providing services both in person and by telemedicine. You will find it at BarnardMedical.org or you can call 202-527-7500.

Bring In Social Support

It is helpful to involve other people in your food adventure. If a family member or friend joins you in your twenty-one-day "test-drive," they can share ideas with you, help with meal planning or food preparation, and be a support at moments of doubt. They will benefit, just as you will.

Sometimes, our families and friends can interfere with healthy changes we are trying to make. That is understandable, because they might be nervous that you will end up taking away their own unhealthy favorite foods. Here are some tips:

- Let your family and friends know that your diet experiment is important to you. Ask that they join you, or, at a minimum, that they not tease you or tempt you with foods you are trying to avoid.
- If you have seriously unhealthful eaters in your household, you might suggest keeping foods on different shelves or in separate parts of the refrigerator.
- Plan a movie night. Cook up some air-popped popcorn and invite your loved ones to watch a film with you. *Forks over Knives*, *What the Health*, and *The Game Changers* are well done, informative, and motivating films about the power of healthful eating.
- As you go along, make extras of food you are preparing for yourself to share with others. It is amazing how naysayers become believers.

You can build extra social support by joining a cooking class in person or remotely, such as a Food for Life class, mentioned above, or listening to nutrition podcasts, such as *The Exam Room*. You will see that millions of people are making the same shifts you are and are learning together in the process.

Bumps in the Road

You will love how you feel when you are fueled by healthful foods. Even so, there are occasional bumps in the road: an unexpected craving, a restaurant dinner where healthful choices are scarce, a family member who is resistant to better foods, and so on. In the sections below, we will look at helpful resources, social support, and other ways to power through whatever challenges might come your way.

LOVE AND LASAGNA

Liz, the research participant we met earlier, had tremendous success with her healthy, plant-based diet. The foods she was eating were tasty and had helped her reach a healthy weight. It was easy to stick with the plan. However, she hit a small bump in the road. She fell in love.

Mr. Right worked on Capitol Hill. He was intelligent, hard-working, and had a good sense of humor. They had worked together on some legal projects when their relationship became more than a work collaboration. Although they had similar tastes in most things, it soon became clear that healthful eating was just not him. He did not challenge Liz's diet at all. But he did not share it, either. When they ate out, it pained her to see him order cheeseburgers, chicken wings, and other foods she had left behind, particularly since he was uncomfortable with his weight. He thought he was stuck with it.

There was only one thing to do: seduce his taste buds. Because he tended to skip breakfast, she made things for him that he could not resist. She had cured herself of her breakfast-neglecting ways and was now hoping to work some magic for him with blueberry muffins, French toast, and waffles with sliced strawberries. She served him veggie sausage, and he did not notice the difference. One day, she tried scrambled tofu with thin strips of grilled tempeh. To her surprise he quite liked both. In fact, it turned out that he was a rather easy sell. As long as he did not have to cook it himself, he liked most everything she made.

As the weeks went by, he noticed that he was losing weight, and he told her that it had to be a result of her cooking. From there, he began to rethink his restaurant choices, too.

One day they were invited to a wedding out of town. His college roommate was getting married. This meant a road trip, plus a wedding reception, which could be tricky for people trying to eat healthfully. However, by this time, Liz was an expert in finding healthy foods on the road. The phrase "Think International" had become her travel motto after having heard our research team use it. Chinese, Italian, Mexican, Indian, and Japanese restaurants were her favorites, and she knew she would always find plenty to eat en route. However, the wedding reception itself was going to be a challenge. She did not want to turn up her nose at whatever was to be served, but she did not want to eat it, either.

While she was mulling over what to do, her boyfriend solved the problem for her. He called his friend—the groom—and, in the course of the conversation, mentioned that Liz was following a vegan diet, and he hoped it would not create any issues for the caterers, since she would be happy with side dishes. His friend reassured him. Lots of people are going in the same direction, he explained, and they had been planning for it. Don't worry, there will be plenty to eat. Sure enough, the evening dinner was a spinach lasagna, and the chef prepared several servings with vegan cheese.

When it was time for toasts, his friend told him, "I see how you are looking at each other. Today is our big day, but let me tell you, *you are next!*"

What If You Are Not Losing Weight Fast Enough?

If weight loss seems slower than you would have expected, here are a few tips.

1. **Check Your BMI.** Sometimes people feel a need to lose weight when they are actually already at a healthy weight

and are simply responding to social pressure. So how do you know if losing weight is a good idea? Check your body mass index. Just search online for a BMI calculator, and plug in your height and weight. If your BMI is between 18.5 and 25.0 kg/m², you are in the healthy range. BMI is not a perfect gauge—some people prefer to be toward the low side or high end within this window, depending on their frame and musculature—but it is a good general guide.

2. **Emphasize the Power Foods.** As you will recall from chapter 2, researchers from Harvard, from our own research team, and from many other centers have identified foods that are most strongly associated with weight loss. Reread chapter 2 to be sure you are taking advantage of the full range of the power foods.

3. **Do a Search-and-Destroy for Fatty Foods.** Jot down the foods you have eaten over the past two days and look for those containing more than trivial amounts of fat: animal products, nuts, nut butters, avocados, or oils. Set these foods aside completely over the next few weeks and see what happens. This often solves the problem.

4. **Check Your Health.** While most people with weight issues do not have an underlying health problem that is making it hard to lose weight, some do. For example, if your thyroid is sluggish, weight loss can be slower. Your doctor can easily check your thyroid function and prescribe treatment, if needed.

Have Foods Become Addicting?

Sometimes our attachment to foods goes beyond taste. Scientists have shown that certain foods can become addicting. Luckily, we have new power to conquer the problem. Here is what you need to know.

First of all, not every food is addictive. You may *like* a crisp apple on a hot summer day, but you never plowed through five of them at a sitting. Similarly, you might *like* grapes or strawberries, but you never stuffed yourself with them to the point of pain. The foods that have addictive power are those that contain compounds that turn on the brain's addictive circuitry. These include cheese, sugar, chocolate, meat, and salty-greasy snacks. Cheese is among the most problematic because it has casomorphins—natural narcotic chemicals that appear to be the basis for its addictive qualities—and a huge calorie load that shows up on the scale. Sugar triggers the release of opiates in the brain, and particularly addictive are foods that mix sugar with some sort of fat—like cookies that combine sugar and butter, or a cake with sugar and shortening. The sugar lures you in, and the fat packs on the unwanted weight.

If food addictions have you in their grip, let me offer some suggestions.

Healthy Substitutions. Nutritional yeast gives you the taste of cheese without the regrets. No, it's not cheese, but it is close enough to the cheesy taste to help you break free.

When it comes to sugar, it is not particularly high in calories—just 4 calories per gram, compared with 9 for butter, shortening, or other fats. So for people aiming to lose weight, one helpful step is to choose cookies or other snacks that are not made with fatty, high-calorie ingredients.

I learned about this during a research study many years ago. We were working with a group of women seeking to lose weight in the years after menopause. They had tried just about every diet you can imagine, including Atkins, South Beach, Jenny Craig, and Nutri-System, and they felt stuck. The study tested a low-fat vegan diet, comparing it with a more conventional diet. For the vegan diet, there were only two rules—avoid animal products and minimize oils. During one of the weekly research meetings where our participants

got together, one of them pointed out that Twizzlers—the red lico-
rice twists sold at convenience stores—have no animal products and
no added oil, and so they met the study requirements perfectly. I
was taken aback, because this was not exactly what I had in mind.
After all, Twizzlers are basically just sugary, starchy, artificially colored junk. However, in research, we set our rules and then have to
live with them, so at that point, we could not rule out Twizzlers or
similar foods.

When the study ended, the average weight loss was thirteen
pounds in fourteen weeks in the vegan group (despite occasional
Twizzlers), and only about eight pounds for the low-calorie diet
group. We then tracked the participants for two additional years,
finding out that the vegan group was able to maintain its weight loss,
while the conventional group regained the lost weight.

The moral of the story is that while sugary candy is not health
food, it may not be the biggest contributor to weight problems.
Rather, the sugar-fat mixtures—fatty cookies, cakes, pies, puddings,
and the like—are much bigger problems.

Before you race out to the convenience store for Twizzlers, let
me encourage you to take a second step. When you are ready, the
next step is to get your dose of sweetness from the foods Mother
Nature had in mind: Fresh fruit is what your taste buds are designed
to detect and, over time, you will come to love it as a dessert and
snack.

Clean Break. In dealing with any addiction, it helps not to tease
yourself with occasional tastes of whatever got you hooked. Many
smokers realize that it is easier to quit completely than to try to limit
themselves to an occasional cigarette. The same is true for most
other addictions. When we try to have a small amount of a problem
food, it reawakens and reinforces our desire for it. But a clean break,
however difficult it may seem at first, uses the power of forgetting.
As time goes by, you discover that you no longer care about whatever
food you were hooked on.

Chuck

Chuck Carroll, host of *The Exam Room* podcast, knows a side of the food world that most people would not want to venture into. As a successful radio host and sports reporter, Chuck worked for major networks and was in demand by radio stations and advertisers alike. But after hours, Chuck had a serious problem with food. At the Taco Bell drive-through, Chuck was not satisfied with a couple of burritos and rice. His typical order consisted of two seven-layer burritos, two beef Grilled Stuft Burritos, one Nachos BellGrande, one chicken quesadilla, one cheesy potato burrito, and a caramel apple empanada. That was 4,370 calories, 196 grams of fat, and 10,420 milligrams of sodium.

This did not start in adulthood. His food addiction was something that had begun in adolescence and worsened over time. Taco Bell was *the* place.

Working as a radio host at a classic rock station and being known as a food lover, he was asked to endorse and follow a "cookie diet" as part of an advertising campaign. For three days, cookies took the place of his daily Taco Bell fix, and he felt truly terrible. He realized he was in fast-food withdrawal and went straight back to his Taco Bell binges. Eventually, Chuck reached 420 pounds, with a size 6X shirt and a sixty-six-inch waist.

Finally, he decided to have bariatric surgery, which made it impossible to eat large portions, at least temporarily. But he knew that, over time, his stomach would likely expand again. So he made a critical decision: to change the way he ate forever. That meant a plant-based diet.

Today, you would not recognize him. Chuck is slim and healthy. He never regained the lost weight, and he has dedicated his life to conveying lifesaving information to others who can benefit. But does he make the occasional trip to the drive-through? Does he sneak a Taco Bell quesadilla here and there? No way. Some people can go to Taco Bell and get a more or less healthy meal. But Chuck would not go there for a glass of water. He has no desire to let the sounds and smells trigger the dysfunctional behavior of years past.

It may be that some people can wrestle an addiction down to something manageable. But for most people, that one moment when you feel you "can handle it" leads to years of regret. If you see part of yourself in Chuck's experience, it pays to avoid temptation.

Overeaters Anonymous. For people with compulsive eating and problems with food, Overeaters Anonymous provides important support. Meetings are in person, online, or over the phone. You can find a meeting near you at OA.org, where you will also find other resources.

HALT. Sometimes cravings arrive out of the blue. But other times there is an identifiable reason for them. People involved in addiction treatment use the acronym "HALT" to recognize common trigger moments. Cravings tend to kick in when we are hungry, angry, lonely, or tired. Recognizing that can help you make sense of them.

The acronym also tells you what to do. When a craving feels overwhelming, let's check:

- If you are hungry, have a healthy snack. No, a banana, apple, or piece of bread may not be what you are really craving, but it takes the edge off hunger and often makes cravings disappear.
- Are you angry or lonely? If so, is there someone you can call, or is there some other healthy way of dealing with it?
- Are you tired? If so, can you close your eyes for a few minutes, take a nap, or plan to go home early?

The HALT method helps enormously, especially at the early stages of breaking free from unhelpful habits.

Healthy Dopamine. All drugs of abuse—alcohol, tobacco, heroin, compulsive gambling, compulsive eating, and, yes, cheese—gain their addictive power because of their effect on dopamine, the brain's pleasure chemical. Whatever other effects drugs may have on your body, they all give you a dopamine boost, which makes you feel better temporarily and keeps you coming back.

Some people tend to have less dopamine activity in their brain cells than other people do, and they are particularly vulnerable to addictions. In the course of our research on diabetes, we have found that about half of people with type 2 diabetes have a genetic trait that causes them to have less dopamine activity than other people.[4] That trait can lead people to overeat as a way to get more dopamine. Then, as weight climbs, diabetes is more likely to strike.

It turns out that you can get dopamine from healthy activities, too. Exercise, social interactions with friends, and even listening to music all stimulate dopamine release in the brain. If you build these into your life, you will have less need to boost dopamine artificially.

Professional Help. Mental health professionals can be very helpful in dealing with compulsive overeating and food addictions. If you go this route, I would encourage you to see a professional who specializes in eating disorders.

The Adventure Begins

You now know more about how foods affect health than most other people. I hope you will share what you have learned with others, and I wish you the best as you put that knowledge to work. Good luck!

MENUS AND RECIPES

SAMPLE MENUS

Day One:

Day Two:

Day Three:

Day Four:

French Toast with Cinnamon Blueberry Syrup   *182; 295*

Loaded Choppy Salad Bowls   *220*

Samosa Lettuce Cups and Mango Dal   *198; 209*

Day Five:

Sheet Pan Chickpea Frittata   *169*

Tofu Tacos   *199*

Quick Stir-Fry and Cucumber Arame Salad   *269; 236*

Day Six:

Tofu Chilaquiles   *178*

Cauliflower BBQ Sliders and Potato Salad   *195; 234*

Red Pepper and Artichoke Paella   *251*

Day Seven:

Blender Oat Waffles with Cinnamon
    Blueberry Syrup   *173; 295*

Convenient Black Bean Burritos with Pinto
    Picnic Salad   *193; 218*

Potato-Lentil Enchiladas with Perfect Brown Rice   *267; 237*

Strawberry Banana Breakfast Bake

SERVES 9   *Easy*

2 tablespoons flax meal

¼ cup water

2 bananas, mashed

1¼ cups unsweetened almond milk

¼ cup unsweetened applesauce

2 teaspoons vanilla extract

2 cups old-fashioned rolled oats

2 teaspoons baking powder

1 teaspoon ground cinnamon

¼ teaspoon sea salt

1 cup chopped strawberries

½ cup sliced strawberries

1 banana, sliced

Maple syrup (optional)

Preheat the oven to 400°F. Line an 8 x 8-inch baking dish with parchment paper so that it overhangs on two sides by an inch or two.

Add the flax and water to a small bowl, whisk to combine, and let sit to thicken for 5 minutes.

In a bowl, mash 2 bananas. Add the milk, applesauce, and vanilla and whisk to combine.

Add the oats, baking powder, cinnamon, and salt to a large bowl and whisk to combine. Add the flax mixture and mashed banana mixture and use a spatula to combine all the ingredients. Fold in the chopped strawberries until evenly dispersed. Transfer to the prepared baking dish.

Top with the sliced strawberries and banana.

Bake for 25 minutes, or until the edges have started to brown and the top appears to have set.

Let cool for 10 minutes before cutting into 9 squares.

PER SERVING (1 SQUARE): 121 CALORIES, 4 G PROTEIN, 19 G CARBOHY-DRATE, 2 G SUGAR, 3 G TOTAL FAT, 2% CALORIES FROM FAT, 0 G SATURATED FAT, 1 G FIBER, 200 MG SODIUM

—DH

Everyday Overnight Oats Three Ways

SERVES 1   *Convenient*

½ cup rolled oats

½ cup unsweetened almond milk

Maple syrup (optional)

ADD-INS:

Triple Berry: Add ⅓ cup frozen triple-berry mix.

Mango and Pear: Add ¼ cup chopped mango and ¼ cup chopped pear.

Apple Cinnamon: Add ½ cup chopped apple with skin removed and ½ teaspoon ground cinnamon.

Add the oats and milk to a small container and stir until well combined.

Add the add-in combo of choice and let the oats sit in the fridge overnight. Make up to 5 days in advance to have your overnight oats ready for an easy breakfast during the week.

PER SERVING (ENTIRE RECIPE WITHOUT ADD-INS): 168 CALORIES, 6 G PRO-TEIN, 28 G CARBOHYDRATE, 1 G SUGAR, 4 G TOTAL FAT, 2% CALORIES FROM FAT, 1 G SATURATED FAT, 4 G FIBER, 3 MG SODIUM

—DH

Sheet Pan Chickpea Frittata

SERVES 8   *Elegant*

1 cup halved cherry tomatoes

½ red pepper, thinly sliced

½ red onion, thinly sliced

1 head broccoli cut into bite-sized florets (3 to 4 cups)

1 (16-ounce) package silken tofu

½ cup unsweetened almond milk

⅔ cup garbanzo bean flour

3 tablespoons nutritional yeast

2 tablespoons cornstarch

1 tablespoon Dijon mustard

1 teaspoon sea salt

1 teaspoon baking powder

½ teaspoon ground turmeric

1 teaspoon kala namak (optional)

1 tablespoon dried rosemary or 2 tablespoons fresh rosemary

Freshly cracked pepper (optional)

Preheat the oven to 350°F. Line a 9 x 13-inch rimmed baking sheet with parchment paper.

Add the tomato, red pepper, onion, and broccoli florets to the baking sheet and bake for 15 minutes, or until the broccoli is fork-tender.

While the vegetables are roasting, add the tofu, milk, flour, nutritional yeast, cornstarch, mustard, salt, baking powder, turmeric, and kala namak, if using, to a blender and blend until smooth and creamy.

Slowly pour the mixture from the blender over the vegetables until it fills the baking sheet. Sprinkle the rosemary evenly over the top and grind some fresh pepper over the top, if using. Return to the oven and bake 24 to 26 minutes, until the mixture appears dry. Remove from the oven and let cool for 10 minutes before slicing.

Cut into 8 squares.

Note: Serve drizzled with White Bean Tzatziki (page 294), Carrot Cauliflower Cheese Sauce (page 290), or Power Greens Pesto (page 292), if desired.

PER SERVING (1 SQUARE): 109 CALORIES, 5 G PROTEIN, 15 G CARBOHY-DRATE, 2 G SUGAR, 2 G TOTAL FAT, 3% CALORIES FROM FAT, 0 G SATURATED FAT, 5 G FIBER, 450 MG SODIUM

—DH

Everything Sweet Potato Sriracha Toast

SERVES 4   *Easy*

2 sweet potatoes

½ teaspoon sea salt

½ teaspoon ground cinnamon

4 pieces whole-grain bread, toasted

Sriracha

Everything bagel seasoning

Preheat the oven to 400°F. Line a baking sheet with parchment paper.

Cut the potatoes in half lengthwise. Place them face down on the prepared baking sheet and bake for 45 to 60 minutes, until they are tender when pierced with a fork. Remove from the oven and let sit until cool enough to handle.

Peel away the skin of the potatoes. Add the potatoes, salt, and cinnamon to a bowl and mash and mix until well combined. Divide the potato mixture among the pieces of toast.

Top with the desired amount of sriracha and everything seasoning.

Note: If you can't find everything bagel seasoning at your local grocer, you can DIY it! In a bowl, mix together 1 tablespoon dried minced garlic, 1 tablespoon dried minced onion, 2 teaspoons black sesame seeds, 2 teaspoons white sesame seeds, and ½ teaspoon Maldon or coarse sea salt. Use as directed in the recipe.

PER SERVING (¼ OF RECIPE): 183 CALORIES, 6 G PROTEIN, 32 G CARBOHYDRATE, 4 G SUGAR, 4 G TOTAL FAT, 2% CALORIES FROM FAT, 1 G SATURATED FAT, 2 G FIBER, 412 MG SODIUM

—*DH*

Green Smoothie Strawberry Pancakes

SERVES 4   *Elegant*

1 cup baby spinach

1½ cups unsweetened almond milk

1 banana, peeled

2½ cups rolled oats

Juice of ½ lemon

2 teaspoons vanilla extract

2 teaspoons baking powder

½ teaspoon ground cinnamon

¼ teaspoon sea salt

1–2 tablespoons maple syrup (optional)

1 cup thinly sliced strawberries

Cinnamon Blueberry Syrup (page 295—optional)

Add the spinach and milk to a blender and blend until smooth and creamy. Add the banana, oats, lemon juice, vanilla, baking powder, cinnamon, and salt. Add the maple syrup at this time, if using as a sweetener. Blend until everything is combined but not smooth. Do not overblend or it will get gummy and sticky. There should still be some texture left from the oats.

Transfer the batter to a bowl and fold in the strawberries.

Heat a large nonstick skillet over medium heat. Pour ⅓ cup of the batter onto the pan for each pancake. Cook until each pancake has bubbles that form across the top, about 3 minutes. Flip and cook on the other side for 3 minutes, or until the edges are dry, and remove from the pan. Top with your favorite fruits and cinnamon blueberry syrup, if using.

PER SERVING (¼ OF RECIPE): 129 CALORIES, 4 G PROTEIN, 22 G CARBOHY-DRATE, 3 G SUGAR, 3 G TOTAL FAT, 3% CALORIES FROM FAT, 0 G SATURATED FAT, 4 G FIBER, 395 MG SODIUM

—DH

Good Morning Greens Smoothie

SERVES 1   *Convenient*

2 cups baby spinach
1 cup frozen strawberries
½ cup unsweetened almond milk
Maple syrup (optional)

Add the spinach, strawberries, and almond milk to a blender. Blend until smooth and creamy.

Sweeten with maple syrup, if desired.

Variations: This is also delicious with frozen mango or a mixture of strawberry and banana, but you could use any fruit you like. Use fresh fruit if desired and add some ice when blending to make it cold. Stick with spinach if you are hoping to have a green smoothie with little to no earthy flavor from the greens.

PER SERVING (ENTIRE RECIPE): 79 CALORIES, 3 G PROTEIN, 16 G CARBOHY-DRATE, 7 G SUGAR, 2 G TOTAL FAT, 3% CALORIES FROM FAT, 0 G SATURATED FAT, 5 G FIBER, 133 MG SODIUM

—DH

Blender Oat Waffles

SERVES 4 *Easy*

3 cups rolled oats

2¼ cups unsweetened nondairy milk

¼ cup silken tofu

1 banana

1 tablespoon baking powder

¼ teaspoon salt

1 tablespoon maple syrup

1 teaspoon vanilla extract

½ teaspoon ground cinnamon

Pinch ground nutmeg

Fresh fruit (optional)

Maple syrup (optional)

Preheat a waffle iron according to manufacturer's instructions.

Add the oats to a high-speed blender and blend into a flour. Add the milk, tofu, banana, baking powder, salt, maple syrup, vanilla, cinnamon, and nutmeg. Blend until smooth and creamy; the batter will be thick.

Lightly spray the waffle iron with cooking spray and follow the manufacturer's instructions to make the waffles.

Batter will thicken more as it sits while you make the waffles; add splashes of water or nondairy milk as needed to loosen it up.

Serve with fresh fruit or maple syrup, if desired.

PER SERVING (¼ OF RECIPE): 132 CALORIES, 7 G PROTEIN, 23 G CARBO-HYDRATE, 4 G SUGAR, 2 G TOTAL FAT, 12% CALORIES FROM FAT, 0 G SATU-RATED FAT, 3 G FIBER, 104 MG SODIUM

—*DH*

British-Style Beans and Greens on Toast

SERVES 4   *Easy*

1 shallot, diced
Water or low-sodium vegetable broth, as needed
1 clove garlic, minced
1 tablespoon tomato paste
1 teaspoon yellow mustard
1 teaspoon apple cider vinegar
1 teaspoon tamari or soy sauce
1 tablespoon maple syrup
1 (15.5-ounce) can low-sodium navy beans, drained and
    rinsed, or 1½ cups cooked navy beans
¼ teaspoon smoked paprika
¼ teaspoon chili powder
2 cups baby spinach
4 pieces whole-grain bread, toasted
Chopped fresh parsley for garnish (optional)
Freshly cracked pepper for garnish (optional)

Heat a nonstick skillet over medium heat. Add the shallot and sauté until soft and translucent. Use 2 tablespoons of water or low-sodium vegetable broth as needed to keep the shallot from sticking. Add the garlic and sauté 1 additional minute, or until fragrant. Add the tomato paste and mix into the garlic and onions; allow the paste to caramelize slightly for a few minutes, stirring frequently to avoid burning. Add liquid as needed.

Add the mustard, vinegar, tamari, and maple syrup and mix to combine. Add the beans, paprika, chili powder, and spinach and mix everything together until well combined. Reduce the heat to low and continue to stir until the beans are heated through and the spinach has wilted completely, about 4 minutes.

Divide the mixture among 4 pieces of toast and sprinkle with chopped fresh parsley and freshly cracked pepper, if using.

PER SERVING (¼ OF RECIPE): 147 CALORIES, 8 G PROTEIN, 30 G CARBOHY-
DRATE, 6 G SUGAR, 1 G TOTAL FAT, 1% CALORIES FROM FAT, 0 G SATURATED
FAT, 8 G FIBER, 149 MG SODIUM

—DH

Cheesy Grits and "Bacon"

SERVES 2 to 3   *Elegant*

Portobello Bacon (page 176)
Barbecue Sauce (page 301—optional)
1 cup water
½ cup grits (or dry polenta)
¼–½ cup soy milk
¼ cup nutritional yeast or vegan cheddar shreds
Salt and pepper
Dash granulated garlic powder (optional)
1–2 green onions, sliced, for garnish (optional)

Prepare portobello bacon and barbecue sauce, if using, and set aside. In a saucepan, bring 1 cup water to a boil. Once the water is boiling, turn off the heat and gradually whisk in the grits, stirring vigorously to avoid lumps. Whisk in additional water to thin further, if desired.

Once grits are ready, gradually stir in the soy milk to cream them up. Stir in the nutritional yeast (or vegan cheese, if using). Season with salt and pepper and garlic powder to taste, if desired. Top grits with sliced green onion, warm portobello bacon, and a drizzle of prepared barbecue sauce, if desired.

Note: Steamed broccoli or kale is a terrific addition. To reheat leftover grits, place in a nonstick saucepan. Add a drizzle of water, soy milk, or vegetable broth. Heat on low, stirring constantly, and breaking up lumps as you stir. Continue cooking until warm.

PER SERVING (½ OF RECIPE): 190 CALORIES, 17 G PROTEIN, 29 G CARBOHY-DRATE, 9 G SUGAR, 2 G TOTAL FAT, 3% CALORIES FROM FAT, 0 G SATURATED FAT, 8 G FIBER, 186 MG SODIUM

—*LN*

Portobello Bacon

SERVES 2 to 4   *Easy*

1–3 teaspoons vegan Worcestershire sauce

1–2 teaspoons pure maple syrup

¼ teaspoon liquid smoke

½ teaspoon granulated garlic powder

½ teaspoon Frank's RedHot sauce (optional)

1 teaspoon low-sodium soy sauce (optional)

4 portobello mushrooms or 16 ounces cremini mushrooms

1–4 tablespoons water or vegetable broth

Salt and pepper (optional)

In a large skillet, whisk together the Worcestershire sauce, maple syrup, liquid smoke, and garlic powder, plus the hot sauce and soy sauce, if using. Set aside.

Remove and discard the stems from the mushrooms. Slice the mushrooms thin or dice them. Add the mushrooms to the skillet and cook over medium heat, stirring regularly, until the mushrooms are tender and start to caramelize, adding water or broth as needed. Season with salt and pepper, if desired.

PER SERVING (¼ OF RECIPE): 5 CALORIES, 0 G PROTEIN, 1 G CARBOHY-DRATE, 1 G SUGAR, 0 G TOTAL FAT, 0% CALORIES FROM FAT, 0 G SATURATED FAT, 2 G FIBER, 74 MG SODIUM

—LN

Personal Pancakes

SERVES 1 *Easy*

1 cup old-fashioned oats
⅔ cup almond milk or other nondairy milk
½ ripe banana or ¼ cup applesauce
Pinch of salt
½ teaspoon vanilla extract
½ teaspoon baking powder
Dash of ground cinnamon (optional)
Cinnamon Blueberry Syrup (page 295) or maple syrup, for
    serving

Prepare the cinnamon blueberry syrup, if using; set aside. In a small blender, blend the oats to form a flour. Add the almond milk, banana, salt, vanilla, and baking powder, plus cinnamon, if using. Blend until smooth but be careful not to overmix or the pancakes will be tough.

Heat a nonstick griddle over medium heat. Once it is warm, pour

⅓ cup batter onto the hot griddle. Once bubbles start to appear, use a flat spatula to flip the pancake. Continue to cook until lightly brown on both sides. Repeat with the remaining batter.

Serve with cinnamon blueberry syrup, maple syrup, or fresh fruit.

Note: Thinner nondairy milks such as almond milk or flax milk work better than creamy milks such as soy milk or oat milk. This recipe can be doubled.

PER SERVING (3 PANCAKES, ENTIRE RECIPE): 212 CALORIES, 7 G PROTEIN, 37 G CARBOHYDRATE, 7 G SUGAR, 5 G TOTAL FAT, 6% CALORIES FROM FAT, 0 G SATURATED FAT, 6 G FIBER, 279 MG SODIUM

—*LN*

Tofu Chilaquiles

SERVES 2   *Easy*

1 (15-ounce) package extra-firm tofu, drained

4 corn tortillas (or store-bought tortilla chips)

¼ cup vegetable broth

½ small onion, diced

2–3 cloves garlic, minced

¼–½ teaspoon ground cumin

¼ teaspoon chili powder

¼–½ cup Enchilada Sauce (page 299) or salsa verde

Salt and pepper (optional)

1–4 tablespoons corn, thawed if frozen, for topping (optional)

Avocado or guacamole, for topping (optional)

Cilantro, for garnish

Lime juice, for topping (optional)

Vegan sour cream (optional)

Hot sauce (optional)

Wrap the tofu in a clean kitchen cloth and place between two cutting boards. Place something heavy on the top board and press the tofu for 20 minutes; unwrap and set it aside. If using corn tortillas, preheat oven to 375°F. Place the tortillas right on the oven rack and bake for 5 to 10 minutes, until crisp. Crumble and set aside. If using store-bought tortilla chips, crumble them and set aside.

Pour ¼ cup broth into a skillet. Add the onions and garlic. Sauté until the onions are translucent. Stir in the spices to coat well. Add the tofu and use a potato masher or fork to break it up into large crumbles. Add the tortilla chips, reserving a few for garnish, if desired. Stir everything together well. Add ¼ cup enchilada sauce and stir to combine.

Heat on low until thoroughly warm and the tortillas have softened slightly. Add additional enchilada sauce, if desired. Add salt and pepper to taste, if desired. Garnish with reserved chips (if any), plus corn, avocado, lime juice, cilantro, vegan sour cream, hot sauce, or other toppings you prefer.

Note: Stale tortillas work terrifically in this recipe. Store-bought New Mexican red chili sauce or taco sauce can be substituted for enchilada sauce. For a "chipotle" version, stir adobo sauce into the enchilada sauce to taste. One (15-ounce) can pinto beans or black beans (drained, rinsed) or refried beans (warmed) is a nice addition to this recipe. A sweet potato can be substituted for the corn chips or tofu; microwave until tender, then dice before adding.

PER SERVING (½ OF RECIPE): 295 CALORIES, 15 G PROTEIN, 56 G CARBOHYDRATE, 3 G SUGAR, 3 G TOTAL FAT, 4% CALORIES FROM FAT, 1 G SATURATED FAT, 11 G FIBER, 185 MG SODIUM

—LN

Mango-Go Smoothie

SERVES 1   *Convenient*

1–3 cups baby spinach

1 cup almond milk

1–4 fresh mint leaves, stemmed

1 cup frozen mango chunks

½ frozen banana

1–2 tablespoons old-fashioned oats

1–3 ice cubes

Juice of 1 small lime (optional)

In a blender, combine the spinach, milk, 1 or 2 mint leaves, mango, banana, and oats with ice. Blend until smooth, adding additional milk or water as needed for desired consistency. Add additional mint to taste, plus lime juice to taste, if using. Serve immediately.

Note: For a sweeter smoothie, add mango juice or sweetener to taste.

PER SERVING (ENTIRE RECIPE): 297 CALORIES, 11 G PROTEIN, 56 G CAR-BOHYDRATE, 40 G SUGAR, 5 G TOTAL FAT, 7% CALORIES FROM FAT, 1 G SATURATED FAT, 7 G FIBER, 151 MG SODIUM

—*LN*

Cajun Grits

SERVES 4 *Elegant*

½ cup vegetable broth (optional)

1 small onion (any variety), diced

1 green bell pepper, diced

1 red bell pepper, diced

1–3 celery stalks, diced

1 (14-ounce) can fire-roasted tomatoes, diced

1–2 tablespoons Cajun seasoning, divided

1 (15-ounce) can lentils or kidney beans, drained and rinsed

½–¾ cup tomato sauce (or ½ teaspoon tomato paste; see note)

Sugar or ketchup (optional)

1 cup grits or dry polenta

3–4 tablespoons nutritional yeast

Salt and pepper (optional)

Vegan sausage (optional)

Louisiana-style hot sauce (optional)

Pour ¼ cup of the vegetable broth or water into a large pot. Add the onions, bell peppers, celery, and diced tomatoes with their juices. Use a spatula to break up any big tomato pieces. Sauté until the onions are translucent. Stir in ½ to 2 teaspoons of the Cajun seasoning to coat. Stir in the lentils and half of the tomato sauce. Heat on low 5 to 10 minutes, until thoroughly warm. Add additional tomato sauce to taste, if desired. If it is too acidic, add 1 to 3 teaspoons of sugar or a squirt of ketchup. Add additional Cajun seasoning to taste, if desired. Set the vegetable-lentil mixture aside.

In a medium pot, bring 4 cups water to a boil. Reduce the heat to low and slowly whisk in the grits. Continue to cook and stir until creamy, 15 to 20 minutes. Stir in the nutritional yeast and 1 to 2 teaspoons of the remaining Cajun seasoning, plus salt and pepper to taste, if desired. Rewarm the vegetable-lentil mixture if needed and prepare the vegan sausage as directed, if using. Serve everything over prepared grits. Drizzle with hot sauce, if using.

Note: 1½ teaspoons tomato paste mixed together with ½ cup water or broth can be used as a substitute for tomato sauce.

PER SERVING (¼ OF RECIPE): 319 CALORIES, 17 G PROTEIN, 62 G CARBOHY-DRATE, 8 G SUGAR, 2 G TOTAL FAT, 2% CALORIES FROM FAT, 0 G SATURATED FAT, 10 G FIBER, 215 MG SODIUM

—LN

French Toast

SERVES 4	*Elegant*

½ baguette or ciabatta

1 cup soy milk

¼ cup chickpea flour (or 2–3 tablespoons cornstarch)

½–1 teaspoon ground cinnamon

Dash of ground nutmeg

1–2 teaspoons pure maple syrup (or ½ very ripe banana)

1 teaspoon vanilla extract (optional)

Pinch of salt (optional)

Dash of nutritional yeast (optional)

Confectioners' sugar, for garnish (optional)

Fresh fruit, for garnish (optional)

Cinnamon Blueberry Syrup (page 295), for garnish (optional)

Maple syrup, for serving

Slice the baguette diagonally into 6 to 8 pieces. If possible, keep slices out overnight to become stale. If using the banana option, blend the banana with soy milk first until well combined. Whisk the soy milk together with the flour, cinnamon, and nutmeg, plus maple syrup, vanilla, salt, and nutritional yeast, if using. Pour the mixture into a shallow bowl; set aside.

Heat a nonstick griddle or flat pan. Dip a bread slice into the wet mixture for 5 to 10 seconds. Place on the heated griddle and cook for about 3 minutes on each side. Repeat the process for each slice.

Garnish with a dusting of confectioners' sugar and fresh fruit or drizzle with cinnamon blueberry syrup. Serve with warmed maple syrup.

Note: Sprouted sandwich breads and heartier multigrain or whole wheat may work, but high-quality thickly sliced breads like baguettes and ciabatta work best. Dip sandwich-style breads very quickly to prevent sogginess. For an even "eggier" appearance and aroma, add a dash (about ⅛ teaspoon) of kala namak and turmeric.

PER SERVING (¼ OF RECIPE): 187 CALORIES, 10 G PROTEIN, 30 G CARBOHY-DRATE, 7 G SUGAR, 3 G TOTAL FAT, 4% CALORIES FROM FAT, 1 G SATURATED FAT, 6 G FIBER, 380 MG SODIUM

—*LN*

Wild Blueberry Muffins

SERVES 12   *Easy*

1 very ripe banana

½ cup nondairy milk

6 ounces vegan yogurt or 3 ounces silken tofu

¼ cup applesauce

¼ teaspoon vanilla or lemon extract (optional)

2 cups whole-wheat pastry flour

1 teaspoon baking powder

½ teaspoon baking soda

Pinch of salt

¼–½ cup vegan sugar

1–4 tablespoons lemon zest or orange zest

1 cup wild blueberries, thawed if frozen

Preheat the oven to 350°F. Line a muffin pan with parchment paper liners or use a nonstick pan. In a blender, combine the banana, milk, yogurt, applesauce, and vanilla, if using. Blend until well combined and set aside. In a mixing bowl, whisk together the flour, baking powder, baking soda, salt, and sugar. Pour in the blended mixture. Stir a few times, then add the citrus zest and blueberries. Stir gently until just combined. If the batter looks too dry, add a splash of non-dairy milk.

Spoon the batter evenly into muffin cups. Bake 15 to 25 minutes, until a toothpick inserted into the center comes out clean. Allow the muffins to cool to room temperature before peeling away liners.

Note: You can use plain, vanilla, lemon, or blueberry-flavored vegan yogurt. If your blueberries are large, toss with a little flour to coat the blueberries first; this will help prevent them from sinking. For a gluten-free version, use Bob's Red Mill Gluten-Free 1:1 Flour mix.

PER SERVING (1 MUFFIN; ¹⁄₁₂ OF RECIPE): 119 CALORIES, 3 G PROTEIN, 25 G CARBOHYDRATE, 8 G SUGAR, 1 G TOTAL FAT, 1% CALORIES FROM FAT, 0 G SATURATED FAT, 3 G FIBER, 82 MG SODIUM

—LN

Perfect Hot Oatmeal

SERVES 1   *Convenient*

½ cup old-fashioned oats
½ cup nondairy milk or water
½ cup water
Pinch of salt (optional)
Maple syrup (optional)
Toppings (e.g., berries, chia seeds; see page 187 for
    suggestions—optional)

In a small saucepan, combine the oats, nondairy milk, and water. Cover and bring to a boil. Reduce the heat to low and simmer, stirring occasionally, 3 to 5 minutes. If the oatmeal becomes too thick, stir in more water or milk. If the oatmeal is too watery, continue to cook uncovered. Remove the oatmeal from the heat and let it rest 1 to 3 minutes. Stir in a pinch of salt, if desired. Add maple syrup (or other sweetener) to taste, if desired. Add any toppings you like before serving. For a creamier oatmeal, stir in a splash of nondairy milk or plain vegan yogurt right before serving.

Note: For a quicker cooking time, soak the oats in the liquid(s) overnight. For a boost of protein, stir in 1 scoop of vegan protein powder once the oatmeal is prepared, plus additional milk or water, as needed.

PER SERVING (ENTIRE RECIPE): 178 CALORIES, 6 G PROTEIN, 29 G CARBO-HYDRATE, 0 G SUGAR, 4 G TOTAL FAT, 1 G SATURATED FAT, 5 G FIBER, 92 MG SODIUM

—*LN*

Perfect Hot Oatmeal with Berries

SERVES 1   *Convenient*

½ cup old-fashioned oats

½ cup nondairy milk or water

½ cup water

½ cup frozen mixed berries

Pinch of salt (optional)

Maple syrup (optional)

Toppings (e.g., berries, chia seeds; see page 187 for suggestions—optional)

In a small saucepan, combine the oats, nondairy milk, and water. Cover and bring to a boil. Reduce the heat to low and simmer 1 to 2 minutes. Add the frozen berries, plus 1 to 2 tablespoons of water. Continue to cook and stir occasionally, 3 to 5 minutes. Remove from the heat and let it rest 1 to 3 minutes. Stir in a pinch of salt, if desired. Add maple syrup (or other sweetener) to taste, if desired. Add any toppings you like before serving.

PER SERVING (ENTIRE RECIPE): 225 CALORIES, 6 G PROTEIN, 39 G CARBO-HYDRATE, 8 G SUGAR, 5 G TOTAL FAT, 1 G SATURATED FAT, 6 G FIBER, 93 MG SODIUM

—*LN*

Perfect Hot Oatmeal with Tea

SERVES 1   *Easy*

1 cup tea (e.g., herbal blueberry tea, chai tea)
½ cup old-fashioned oats
Pinch of salt (optional)
Maple syrup (optional)
Toppings (e.g., berries, chia seeds—optional)

Prepare the tea as directed (see package) in 1 cup of water. Discard the tea bag. In a small saucepan, combine the oats and prepared tea. Cover and bring to a boil. Reduce the heat to low and simmer, stirring occasionally, 3 to 5 minutes. If the oatmeal becomes too thick, stir in additional water or nondairy milk. If the oatmeal is too watery, continue to cook uncovered. Remove from the heat and let it rest 1 to 3 minutes. Stir in a pinch of salt, if desired. Add maple syrup (or other sweetener) to taste, if desired. Add any toppings you like before serving.

Note: For a quicker cooking time, soak oats in the liquid(s) overnight. For a creamier oatmeal, stir in a splash of nondairy milk or plain vegan yogurt right before serving.

OATMEAL TOPPING SUGGESTIONS:

Any of the above oatmeal variations can be topped with sliced banana, diced apple, diced pear, fresh or frozen berries (e.g., raspberries, blueberries, blackberries, strawberries), raw nuts (e.g., chopped walnuts, crushed pecans), a tablespoon of peanut butter or almond butter, a sprinkling of ground flaxseeds, chia seeds, hemp seeds, or dried fruit (e.g., raisins, chopped apricots). You can also add a few dashes of ground cinnamon, ground cardamom, or pumpkin pie spice, a light drizzle of maple syrup, a tablespoon of fruit-flavored jam or jelly, brown sugar, a dollop of vegan yogurt, or, for a savory option, sriracha and sliced green onions.

PER SERVING (ENTIRE RECIPE): 155 CALORIES, 3 G PROTEIN, 28 G CARBO-HYDRATE, 0 G SUGAR, 3 G TOTAL FAT, 3% CALORIES FROM FAT, 1 G SATU-RATED FAT, 4 G FIBER, 2 MG SODIUM

—*LN*

Grilled Tofu

SERVES 8   *Easy*

1 (15-ounce) package firm tofu
1 teaspoon ground ginger
1 tablespoon nutritional yeast flakes
4 tablespoons soy sauce

Slice the tofu into 8 short strips. Fry in a nonstick pan until brown, turning once. Serve on a plate topped with ginger, nutritional yeast, and soy sauce.

PER SERVING (1 STRIP): 51 CALORIES, 5 G PROTEIN, 2 G CARBOHYDRATE, 0 G SUGAR, 3 G TOTAL FAT, 53% CALORIES FROM FAT, 0 G SATURATED FAT, 1 G FIBER, 268 MG SODIUM

—*NB*

Grilled Tempeh

SERVES 4 *Easy*

1 (8-ounce) package tempeh
4 tablespoons soy sauce

Slice the tempeh crosswise into 4 sections, then slice each section into 2 thin wafer-like strips. Dip each briefly into the soy sauce, then fry in a nonstick skillet until brown and crispy, turning once. If there is moisture left after cooking, place the cooked tempeh strips on a paper towel and microwave for 30 to 60 seconds to let the moisture evaporate.

PER SERVING (2 STRIPS): 115 CALORIES, 13 G PROTEIN, 9 G CARBOHY-DRATE, 0 G SUGAR, 3 G TOTAL FAT, 23% CALORIES FROM FAT, 0 G SATURATED FAT, 4 G FIBER, 511 MG SODIUM

—*NB*

Creamy Spinach and Artichoke Wraps

SERVES 4 *Easy*

1 (15.5-ounce) can low-sodium cannellini or great northern
   beans, drained and rinsed, or 1½ cups cooked beans

¼ cup water

Juice of ½ lemon

¼ cup nutritional yeast

2 cloves garlic

1 teaspoon onion powder

1 teaspoon sea salt

1 (14-ounce) can artichoke hearts, drained, rinsed, and lightly
   chopped

2 cups baby spinach

4 large low-sodium whole-wheat tortillas

Balsamic vinegar (optional)

Sun-dried tomatoes (not packed in oil), chopped or julienned
   (optional)

Add the beans, water, lemon juice, nutritional yeast, garlic, onion powder, and salt to a food processor. Blend until smooth and creamy. Add the artichokes to the bean mixture and pulse to combine. Do not puree the artichokes; there should still be chunks of artichoke in the mixture.

Divide the spinach among the tortillas and top with the bean-artichoke mixture. Add a drizzle of balsamic vinegar and sun-dried tomatoes, if desired.

Tuck in both ends of the tortilla and roll it up tightly, being careful not to split the tortilla.

Note: Serve the bean-artichoke mixture as a dip with your favorite vegetables or crisps. Additionally, it can be used to top a green salad.

PER SERVING (1 WRAP): 206 CALORIES, 12 G PROTEIN, 40 G CARBOHYDRATE, 1 G SUGAR, 0 G TOTAL FAT, 1% CALORIES FROM FAT, 0 G SATURATED FAT, 5 G FIBER, 598 MG SODIUM

—DH

Mediterranean Chickpea Salad Sandwiches

SERVES 4   *Easy*

1 (15.5-ounce) can low-sodium chickpeas, drained and
    rinsed, or 1½ cups cooked chickpeas

1 Roma tomato, seeds removed, and small-diced

¾ cup small-diced red onion

½ cup chopped roasted red pepper, drained from a jar

2 tablespoons roughly chopped capers

1 tablespoon finely chopped fresh dill or 1 teaspoon dried dill

1 teaspoon dried basil

¼ teaspoon sea salt

Juice of ½ lemon

8 slices low-sodium whole-wheat bread, toasted

4 leaves romaine lettuce

24 thin slices of cucumber

½ cup White Bean Tzatziki (page 294—optional)

Add the chickpeas to a bowl and smash with a fork. Add the tomato, onion, red pepper, capers, dill, basil, sea salt, and lemon juice and mix to combine.

Build a sandwich starting with a piece of bread topped with a leaf of romaine, add ¼ of the chickpea mixture, 6 cucumber slices, and top with 2 tablespoons tzatziki, if using. Top with another piece of bread. Make 3 more sandwiches with the remaining ingredients.

PER SERVING (¼ OF RECIPE): 322 CALORIES, 13 G PROTEIN, 61 G CARBOHY-DRATE, 3 G SUGAR, 4 G TOTAL FAT, 2% CALORIES FROM FAT, 1 G SATURATED FAT, 10 G FIBER, 352 MG SODIUM

—DH

Buffalo Cauliflower and Hummus Wraps

SERVES 4   *Easy*

4 cups cauliflower (1 head), cut into small bite-sized florets

¼ cup Frank's RedHot sauce

2 tablespoons nutritional yeast

½ teaspoon garlic powder

½ teaspoon onion powder

¼ teaspoon sea salt

1 cup Classic Oil-Free Hummus (page 293) or store-bought hummus

2 cups shredded romaine lettuce

1 cup shredded carrots

4 large low-sodium whole-wheat tortillas

Preheat the oven to 425°F. Line a baking sheet with parchment paper.

Cut the florets to a uniform size so they cook evenly.

Add the cauliflower to a bowl with the hot sauce and toss to coat the cauliflower. Add the nutritional yeast, garlic powder, onion powder, and salt. Toss to combine and coat all of the pieces of cauliflower with the spices. Transfer the cauliflower to the prepared baking sheet.

Bake for 15 minutes, then toss and bake an additional 10 minutes, or until the cauliflower appears dry and is fork-tender.

Divide the hummus, lettuce, carrots, and cauliflower among the tortillas. Tuck in both ends of the tortilla and roll it up tightly, being careful not to split the tortilla.

PER SERVING (¼ OF RECIPE): 195 CALORIES, 11 G PROTEIN, 42 G CARBOHYDRATE, 5 G SUGAR, 7 G TOTAL FAT, 3% CALORIES FROM FAT, 1 G SATURATED FAT, 7 G FIBER, 525 MG SODIUM

—DH

Brussels Sprout and Pinto Tacos
with Mango Salsa

SERVES 4　　　　　　　　　　　　　　　　　　　　　　*Elegant*

4 cups shredded brussels sprouts
1 (15.5-ounce) can low-sodium pinto beans, drained and
　　rinsed, or 1½ cups cooked pinto beans
1 tablespoon reduced-sodium taco seasoning
1 cup Mango Salsa (page 302)
8 (6-inch) corn tortillas
Creamy Tofu Sauce (page 304), for garnish (optional)
Scallions, thinly sliced, for garnish (optional)
Edible flowers or microgreens, for garnish (optional)

Heat a large nonstick skillet over medium heat. Add the brussels sprouts, pinto beans, and taco seasoning to the skillet and sauté for 4 to 6 minutes, until the brussels sprouts have cooked down in size.

Add 2 tablespoons of water or vegetable broth to prevent the brussels sprouts from sticking; add more liquid as needed.

Divide the mixture among taco shells and top with the mango salsa. Garnish with the tofu sauce, scallions, edible flowers, or microgreens, if using.

PER SERVING (¼ OF RECIPE): 271 CALORIES, 10 G PROTEIN, 48 G CARBOHYDRATE, 12 G SUGAR, 5 G TOTAL FAT, 2% CALORIES FROM FAT, 1 G SATURATED FAT, 10 G FIBER, 457 MG SODIUM

—DH

Convenient Black Bean Burritos

SERVES 4 *Convenient*

1 (15.5-ounce) can low-sodium black beans, drained and rinsed, or 1½ cups cooked black beans
½ cup store-bought salsa
¼ teaspoon ground cumin
¼ teaspoon garlic powder
¼ teaspoon onion powder
Sea salt, to taste
4 large low-sodium whole-wheat tortillas

Add the black beans and salsa to a pot, stir to combine, and heat over medium heat. Continue stirring until the mixture starts to simmer; add the cumin, garlic powder, and onion powder and stir to combine. Continue to cook until everything is heated all the way through. Taste and season with salt, if desired. Remove from the heat.

Divide the mixture among 4 tortillas, tuck the sides in, and roll up into a tight burrito. Serve immediately or wrap in plastic wrap or aluminum foil and freeze.

If freezing, to reheat, remove the burrito from its wrapper and microwave for 3 minutes, then flip and microwave for an additional 3 minutes. Alternatively, you can bake at 425°F for 25 minutes, or until the burrito is heated through.

Note: Add vegetables! Heat a large nonstick skillet over medium-high heat. Sauté your favorite vegetables in the skillet. When the vegetables are sautéed to your liking, continue with the recipe as written by adding the beans, salsa, cumin, garlic powder, onion powder, and salt and letting the mixture cook for 2 to 4 minutes, until heated through. You can also add rice and spinach to this; cook long enough to wilt the spinach down and heat the rice all the way through.

PER SERVING (1 BURRITO): 323 CALORIES, 14 G PROTEIN, 55 G CARBOHY-DRATE, 3 G SUGAR, 5 G TOTAL FAT, 2% CALORIES FROM FAT, 1 G SATURATED FAT, 14 G FIBER, 589 MG SODIUM

—DH

Weeknight Bean Burgers

SERVES 4   *Easy*

1 (15-ounce) can black beans or kidney beans, drained and rinsed

2 tablespoons ketchup

1 tablespoon prepared yellow mustard

1 teaspoon granulated onion powder

1 teaspoon granulated garlic powder

5 tablespoons instant oats

Salt or hot sauce (optional)

4 hamburger buns

Burger toppings (e.g., lettuce, tomato, vegan cheese, pickles)

Preheat the oven to 400°F and line a baking sheet with parchment paper and set aside. In a mixing bowl, mash the beans with a fork until coarse and only some half beans remain. Stir in the ketchup, mustard, and spices and mix well. Stir in the oats. Add salt or hot sauce to taste, if desired.

For best results, refrigerate the mixture for 5 to 30 minutes. Divide the mixture into 4 equal portions and use your hands to shape into tight patties. Place the patties on a baking sheet. Bake 10 minutes, then flip. Bake for another 5 minutes, or until just crisp on the outside. Serve on buns with your favorite burger toppings.

PER SERVING (¼ OF RECIPE; 1 BURGER, EXCLUDING TOPPINGS): 227 CALORIES, 10 G PROTEIN, 40 G CARBOHYDRATE, 6 G SUGAR, 3 G TOTAL FAT, 4% CALORIES FROM FAT, 1 G SATURATED FAT, 5 G FIBER, 291 MG SODIUM

—*LN*

Cauliflower BBQ Sliders

SERVES 4 *Easy*

1–1¼ cups Barbecue Sauce (page 301) or store-bought sauce
1 head cauliflower
Salt and pepper (optional)
Creamy Coleslaw (page 230—optional)
4 hamburger buns

Prepare the barbecue sauce, if using the recipe, and set aside. Preheat the oven to 350°F and set aside a 12 x 9-inch rectangular glass baking dish. Cut the cauliflower into florets and discard stems. Toss the florets with barbecue sauce until well coated.

Transfer the florets to the baking dish along with any loose sauce. Bake for 30 minutes.

Stir well, then use a potato masher, firm spatula, or a fork to break apart the cauliflower. Repeat the process one to two more times for a total bake time of 60 to 90 minutes, until the cauliflower reaches the desired tenderness. Leave the cauliflower as chunky or as mashed up as you like.

Season with salt and pepper, if desired. While the cauliflower is cooking, prepare the coleslaw, if using. Serve the mashed barbecue cauliflower on buns. Top with coleslaw, if using.

Note: For a quicker cooking time, blanch the entire head of cauliflower in a pot of boiling water for a couple of minutes and then crumble and roast at 425°F for 20 minutes, or until crispy.

4 SLIDERS: 239 CALORIES, 6 G PROTEIN, 49 G CARBOHYDRATE, 19 G SUGAR, 2 G TOTAL FAT, 3% CALORIES FROM FAT, 1 G SATURATED FAT, 5 G FIBER, 474 MG SODIUM

—*LN*

Mushroom Quesadillas

SERVES 4   *Easy*

1 cup Classic Oil-Free Hummus (page 293) or store-bought
    hummus
¼ cup vegetable broth
1 tablespoon low-sodium soy sauce
¼–1 teaspoon chili powder
8 ounces brown mushrooms, stemmed and sliced
2–6 tablespoons diced onion (optional)
4 cups baby spinach
4 large tortillas (or wraps)
1 sliced roasted red bell pepper (optional)
Toppings (e.g., salsa, guacamole, vegan sour
    cream—optional)

Prepare the hummus and set aside. Pour the broth into a skillet. Stir in the soy sauce and chili powder. Add the mushrooms and the diced onion, if using. Sauté until the mushrooms are very tender and most of the liquid has cooked off. Add the spinach and stir until it softens and all of the liquid has evaporated. Turn off the heat and set aside briefly.

Spread the hummus on top of an entire tortilla. Place the mushroom mixture on half of the tortilla. Add a few bell pepper strips, if using, on top of the cooked mushrooms. If using guacamole, spoon on top of mushrooms and peppers or leave for garnish. Fold the empty side of the tortilla over on top of the mushrooms and peppers to make a "quesadilla."

Toast the quesadilla in a dry nonstick skillet for 3 to 4 minutes on each side, until warm and crisp. Repeat the process. Serve quesadillas with salsa, guacamole, and vegan sour cream, if using.

Note: Spicy flavored hummus (e.g., chipotle flavored), red pepper hummus, black olive hummus, garlic hummus, cilantro-jalapeño hummus, and roasted garlic hummus all create lovely, subtle variations.

PER SERVING (¼ OF RECIPE): 177 CALORIES, 9 G PROTEIN, 23 G CARBOHYDRATE, 2 G SUGAR, 7 G TOTAL FAT, 9% CALORIES FROM FAT, 1 G SATURATED FAT, 7 G FIBER, 496 MG SODIUM

—LN

Samosa Lettuce Cups

SERVES 2   *Elegant*

Creamy Garlic Yogurt Sauce (page 306—optional)

3 small russet potatoes or 5 red potatoes

¼–½ cup vegetable broth

1–3 tablespoons soy milk (optional)

¼ cup diced onion

1–2 small carrots, diced

1½ teaspoons mild yellow curry powder

¾–1 cup canned lentils or chickpeas, drained and rinsed

½ cup frozen peas

1–2 tablespoons ketchup (optional)

Juice of ½ lemon

Salt and pepper

1 head romaine heart lettuce

Cilantro, for garnish (optional)

Prepare the creamy garlic yogurt sauce, if using, and set aside to chill. Boil or pressure-cook the potatoes. Remove the potato skins, if desired. Mash the cooked potatoes well, adding cooking water, vegetable broth, or soy milk as needed to create a creamy mashed potato consistency; set aside.

Pour ¼ cup broth into a skillet. Sauté the onions until translucent. Add the carrots and curry powder plus additional broth, if needed. Continue to cook until the carrots are fork-tender. Stir in the lentils, peas, and mashed potatoes. Mix well and cook until thoroughly warmed, stirring regularly.

Taste, adding ketchup for a hint of sweetness, if desired. Squeeze the lemon juice over the top and stir in. Add salt and pepper to taste. Spoon the potato filling into the lettuce cups. Garnish with cilantro, if desired. Serve with prepared creamy garlic yogurt sauce, if using.

Note: You can substitute ½ teaspoon ground cumin, 1 teaspoon garam masala, a dash of ground ginger, or a dash of ground turmeric (for color) for the curry powder.

PER SERVING (½ OF RECIPE): 300 CALORIES, 13 G PROTEIN, 64 G CARBOHYDRATE, 7 G SUGAR, 1 G TOTAL FAT, 1% CALORIES FROM FAT, 0 G SATURATED FAT, 16 G FIBER, 81 MG SODIUM

—*LN*

Tofu Tacos

SERVES 4   *Elegant*

1 (14-ounce) package extra-firm tofu, drained

1½ tablespoons taco seasoning

1 tablespoon Bragg Liquid Aminos (or soy sauce)

1–2 teaspoons prepared yellow mustard

1½ tablespoons ketchup or ¼ cup traditional salsa

½ teaspoon dried oregano

½ teaspoon ground cumin

¼ teaspoon smoked paprika

2 teaspoons nutritional yeast

1–2 teaspoons vegan Worcestershire sauce (optional)

6 taco shells or corn tortillas

2–3 cups shredded lettuce

1 diced tomato

Vegan cheese shreds (optional)

Guacamole (optional)

Wrap the tofu in a clean kitchen towel and place it between two cutting boards. Add something heavy onto the top board to press the tofu for 20 minutes.

Unwrap and freeze the pressed tofu overnight or until solid. Thaw the tofu completely and squeeze out any excess water. Crumble the tofu into a mixing bowl. Add the taco seasoning, liquid aminos, mustard, ketchup, spices, and nutritional yeast and mix well. Stir in the Worcestershire sauce, if using.

For best results, let the tofu mixture "marinate" in the fridge for several hours or overnight again. Preheat the oven to 400°F and line a baking sheet with parchment paper. Spread the seasoned tofu out evenly. Bake 20 to 30 minutes, until crisp but not hard, flipping halfway.

Spoon the crumbles into the taco shells. Add shredded lettuce and diced tomato on top, plus vegan cheese and guacamole, if using.

PER SERVING (¼ OF RECIPE): 293 CALORIES, 12 G PROTEIN, 33 G CARBOHYDRATE, 4 G SUGAR, 3 G TOTAL FAT, 17% CALORIES FROM FAT, 3 G SATURATED FAT, 4 G FIBER, 583 MG SODIUM

—LN

Faux Tuna Sandwiches

SERVES 4	Easy

½ teaspoon onion flakes or 1–2 tablespoons finely chopped red onion

1 (15-ounce) can chickpeas, drained and rinsed

1–3 tablespoons vegan mayonnaise (or yogurt)

1 celery stalk, finely chopped

1–2 tablespoons finely chopped dill pickle or dill relish

1–3 teaspoons low-sodium soy sauce

2 teaspoons nutritional yeast

½ teaspoon kelp granules (optional; for a fishier taste)

Black pepper

8 slices whole-grain bread

If using fresh red onion, soak it in cold water 5 minutes, then drain and set aside. In a mixing bowl, mash the chickpeas with a fork or, alternatively, pulse the chickpeas in a food processor until coarse.

Stir together the mashed chickpeas with the onion, 1 tablespoon mayonnaise, celery, dill pickle, soy sauce, nutritional yeast, and kelp, if using, plus several dashes of black pepper, or to taste. Add additional mayonnaise if needed or desired. Serve on bread to make sandwiches.

Any of the following items can be added to make it your own: finely chopped green apple (about ¼ cup); flat-leaf parsley; Dijon mustard and lemon juice (about 2 teaspoons each); whole-grain mustard (1 tablespoon); Dijon mustard (1 tablespoon) and sweet pickle relish (2 tablespoons); hot sauce (e.g., Cholula); or vegan Parmesan cheese (about 1 tablespoon).

Note: You can substitute 1 (8-ounce) package of tempeh for the chickpeas. Boil the tempeh in water 10 minutes, then drain, cool, and crumble or shred. Proceed as directed.

PER SERVING (¼ OF RECIPE): 235 CALORIES, 12 G PROTEIN, 42 G CARBO-
HYDRATE, 8 G SUGAR, 4 G TOTAL FAT, 5% CALORIES FROM FAT, 9 G FIBER,
578 MG SODIUM

—LN

Creamy Chipotle Butternut Soup

SERVES 8   *Elegant*

1 large butternut squash (2.5–3 lbs.), peeled and cut into
    1-inch cubes

1 onion, diced

2 tablespoons water or vegetable broth, as needed

4 cloves garlic, minced

1–2 chipotle chilies in adobo sauce, chopped; start with 1
    and add more if you want spicier soup

1–2 tablespoons sauce from chili adobo, start with 1 and add
    more if you want spicier soup

1 teaspoon smoked paprika

1 teaspoon ground cumin

1 teaspoon dried oregano

1½ teaspoons sea salt

¼ teaspoon ground black pepper

4 cups low-sodium vegetable broth

Juice of 1 lime

Creamy Tofu Sauce (page 304—optional)

Oil-Free Crispy Chickpea Croutons (page 296), for garnish (optional)

Scallion, thinly sliced, for garnish (optional)

Preheat the oven to 425°F. Line a baking sheet with parchment paper.

Add the cubes of squash to the prepared baking sheet and roast for 30 minutes, or until tender when pierced with a fork. Remove from the oven and set aside.

Heat a large stockpot over medium heat. Add the onion and sauté 4 minutes, or until translucent. Add 2 tablespoons of water or vegetable broth as needed to prevent the onion from sticking. Add the garlic and chipotle chilies and sauté 1 additional minute, or until fragrant; add liquid as needed. Add the adobo sauce, paprika, cumin, oregano, salt, pepper, vegetable broth, and lime juice and stir to combine. Turn off the heat.

Use an immersion blender and blend until smooth and creamy. Alternatively, transfer to a blender and blend until smooth and creamy. Taste for spice level at this time and add more chilies and adobo sauce, if desired.

Serve in bowls garnished with creamy tofu sauce, croutons, and scallions, if desired.

PER SERVING (1¼ CUPS): 90 CALORIES, 2 G PROTEIN, 21 G CARBOHYDRATE, 5 G SUGAR, 0 G TOTAL FAT, 0% CALORIES FROM FAT, 0 G SATURATED FAT, 4 G FIBER, 539 MG SODIUM

—DH

Very Fast Veggie Lentil Soup

SERVES 8   *Easy*

1 onion, diced

2 celery stalks, thinly sliced

2 carrots, peeled and thinly sliced

4 cloves garlic, minced

6 cups low-sodium vegetable broth

1 russet potato, skin on, cut into ½-inch cubes

1 cup corn, frozen or fresh

1 head broccoli, cut into tiny bite-sized florets

2 (15.5-ounce) cans low-sodium brown lentils, drained and
    rinsed, or 3 cups cooked brown lentils

1 (14.5 ounce) can no-salt-added diced tomatoes, with juices

1½ cups kale, roughly chopped into small pieces

1 teaspoon dried oregano

1 teaspoon sea salt

½ teaspoon black pepper

Heat a large stockpot over medium heat. Add the onion, celery, and carrots and sauté for 3 minutes, or until the onions are soft. Add the garlic and sauté 1 additional minute, or until fragrant.

Add the broth and potato, then cover and bring to a boil. Reduce to a simmer and continue to cook, covered, for 6 to 8 minutes, until the potatoes are fork-tender. Add the corn, broccoli, lentils, tomatoes, kale, oregano, salt, and pepper and let simmer for 2 to 4 minutes, covered, until the broccoli has become fork-tender.

PER SERVING (1½ CUPS): 169 CALORIES, 9 G PROTEIN, 33 G CARBOHY-DRATE, 6 G SUGAR, 1 G TOTAL FAT, 1% CALORIES FROM FAT, 0 G SATURATED FAT, 9 G FIBER, 482 MG SODIUM

—DH

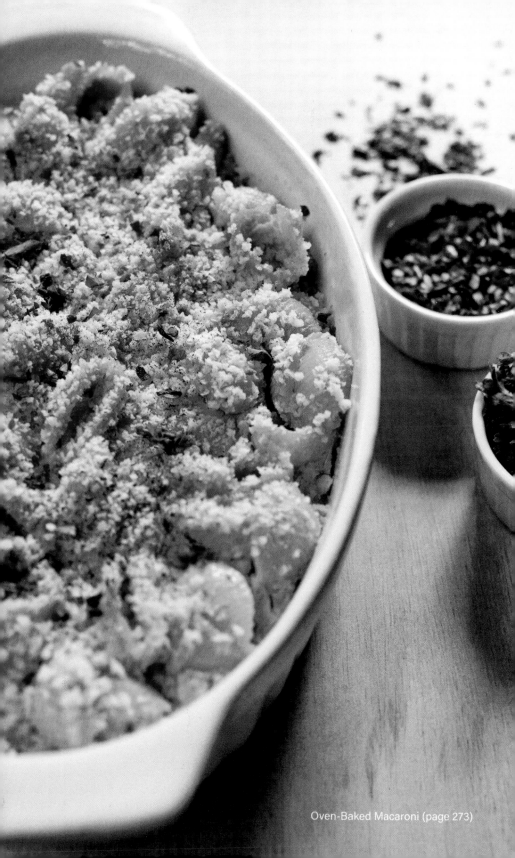

Oven-Baked Macaroni (page 273)

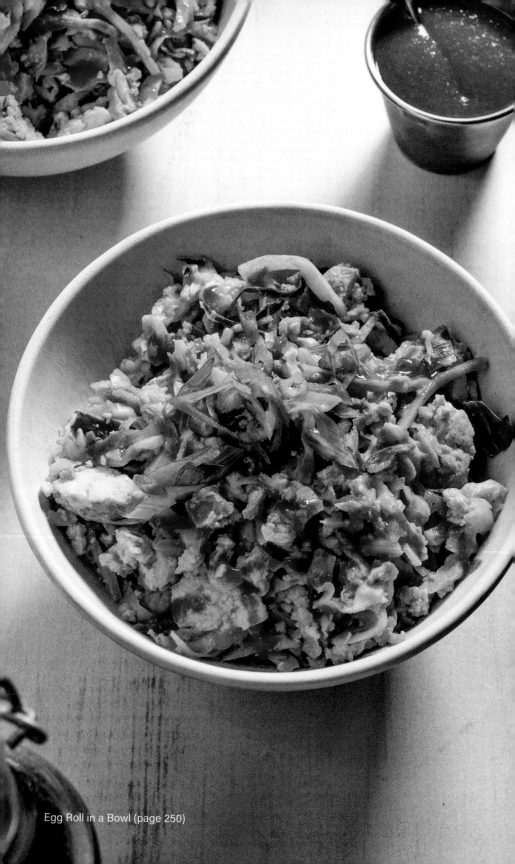

Egg Roll in a Bowl (page 250)

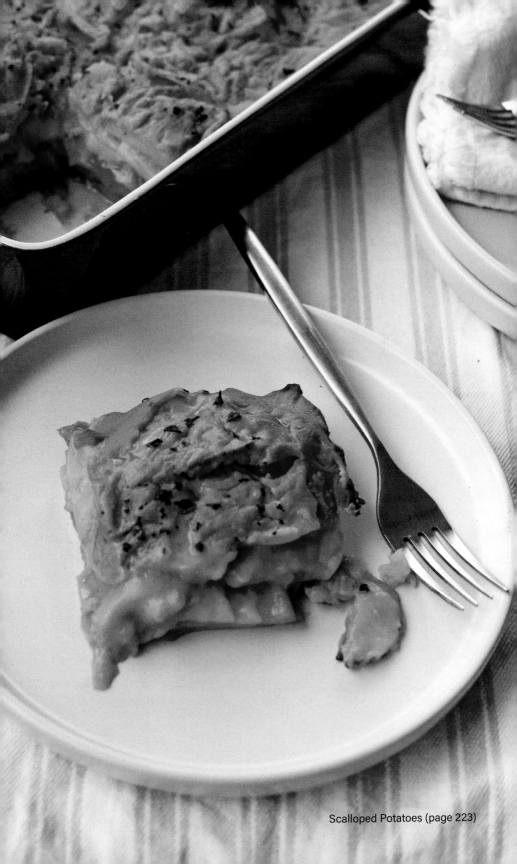

Scalloped Potatoes (page 223)

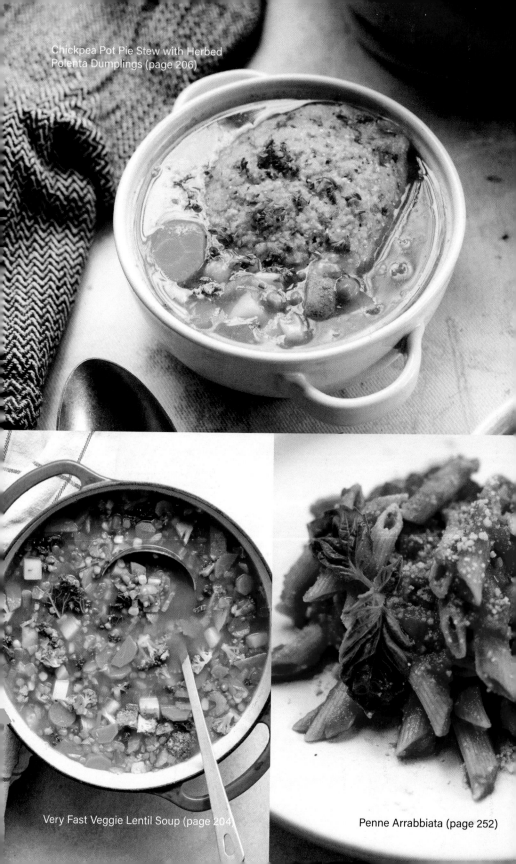

Chickpea Pot Pie Stew with Herbed Polenta Dumplings (page 206)

Very Fast Veggie Lentil Soup (page 204)

Penne Arrabbiata (page 252)

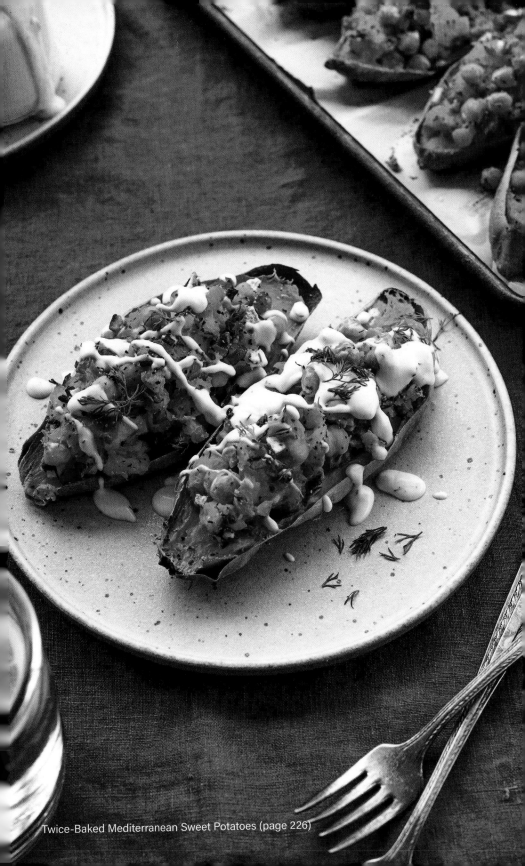

Twice-Baked Mediterranean Sweet Potatoes (page 226)

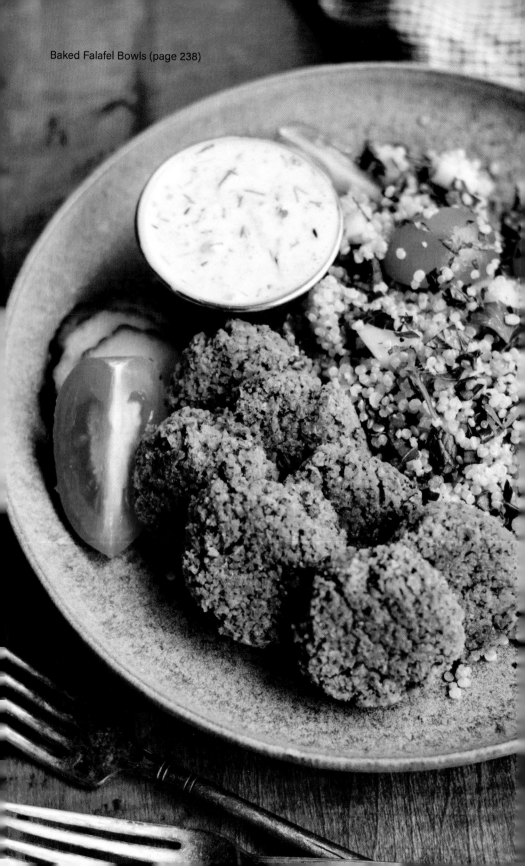

Baked Falafel Bowls (page 238)

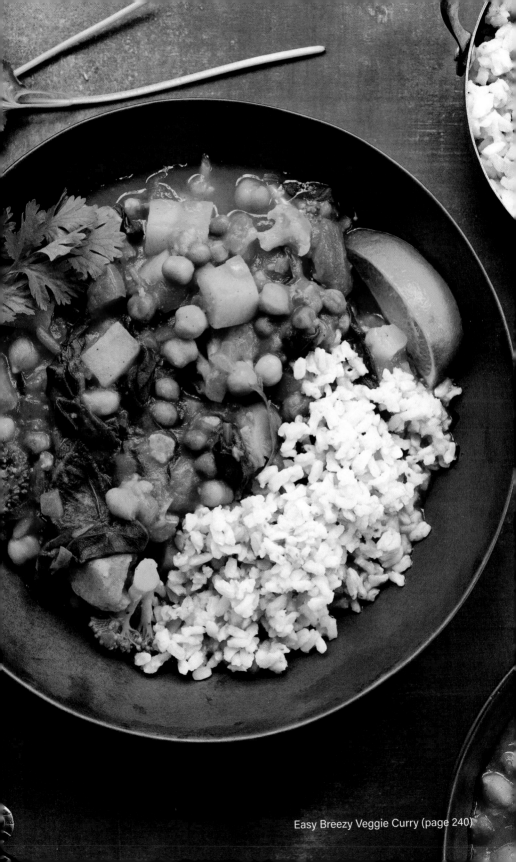

Easy Breezy Veggie Curry (page 240)

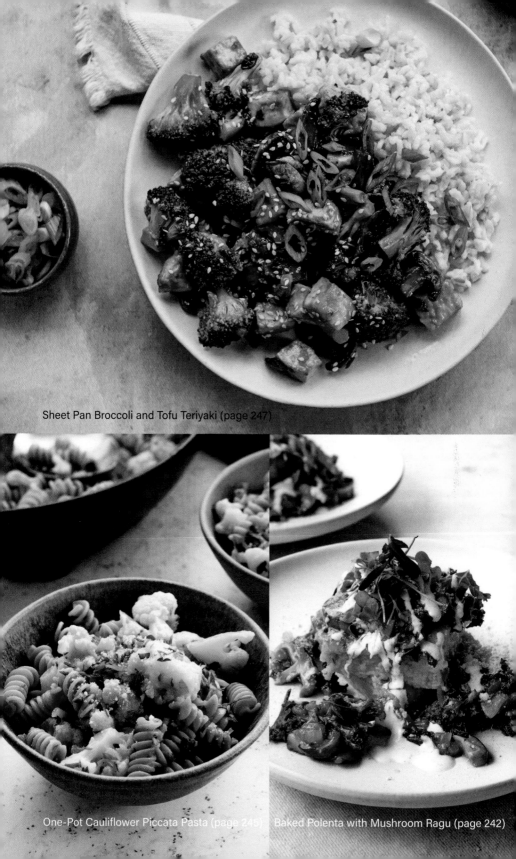

Sheet Pan Broccoli and Tofu Teriyaki (page 247)

One-Pot Cauliflower Piccata Pasta (page 245)

Baked Polenta with Mushroom Ragu (page 242)

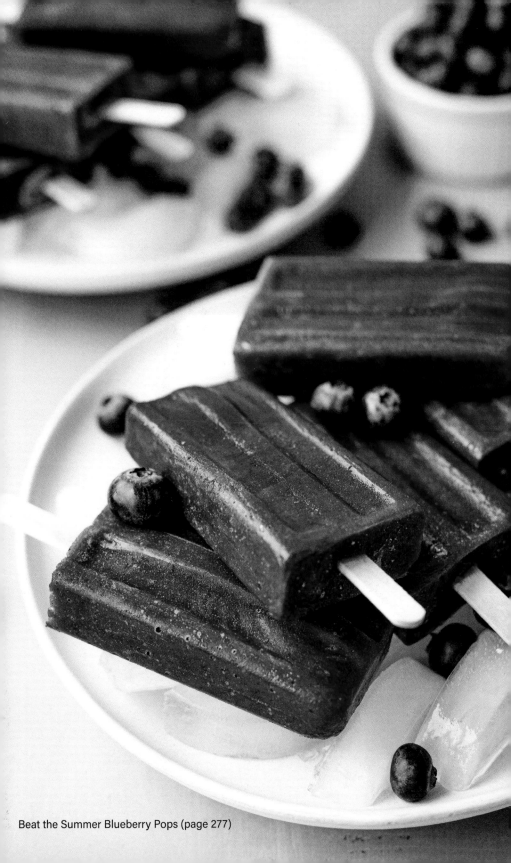

Beat the Summer Blueberry Pops (page 277)

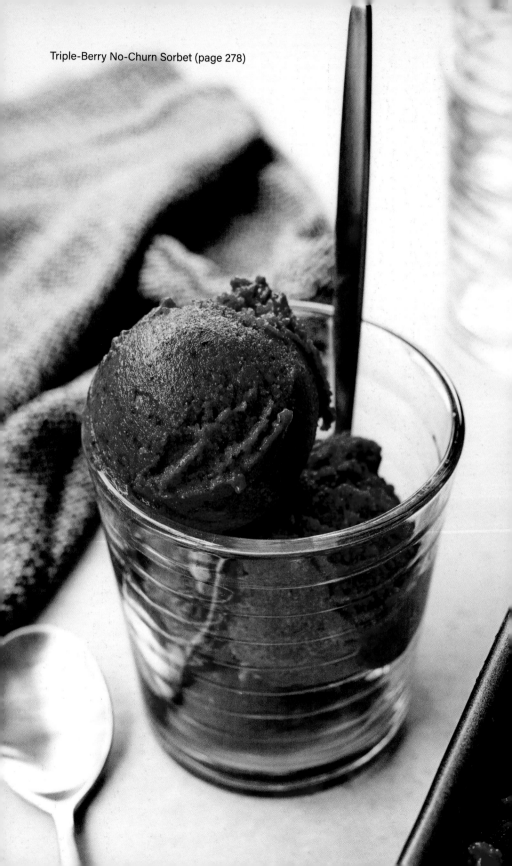

Triple-Berry No-Churn Sorbet (page 278)

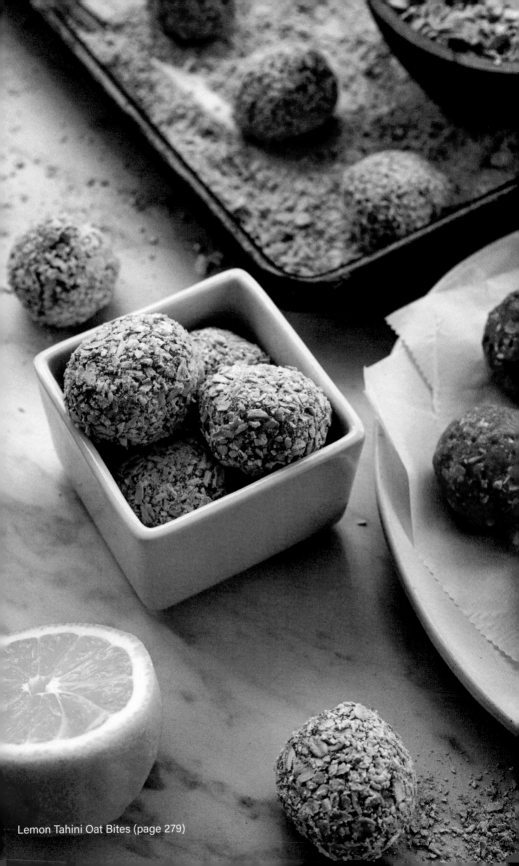

Lemon Tahini Oat Bites (page 279)

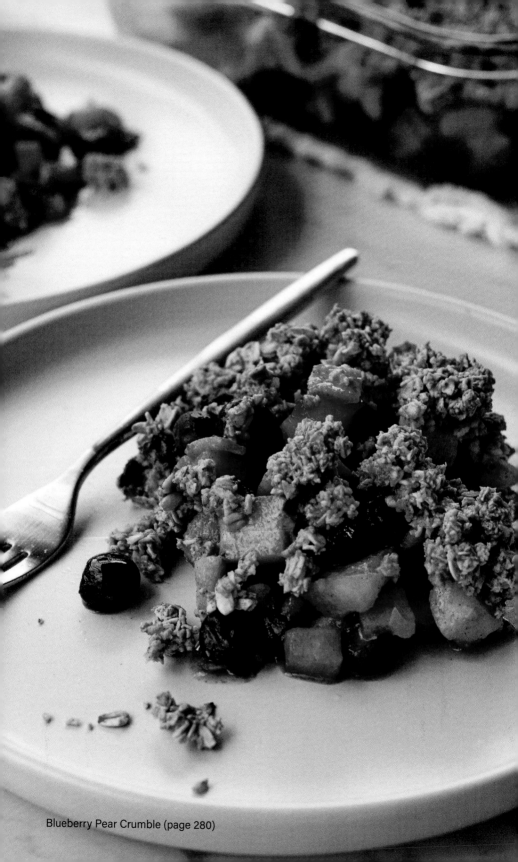

Blueberry Pear Crumble (page 280)

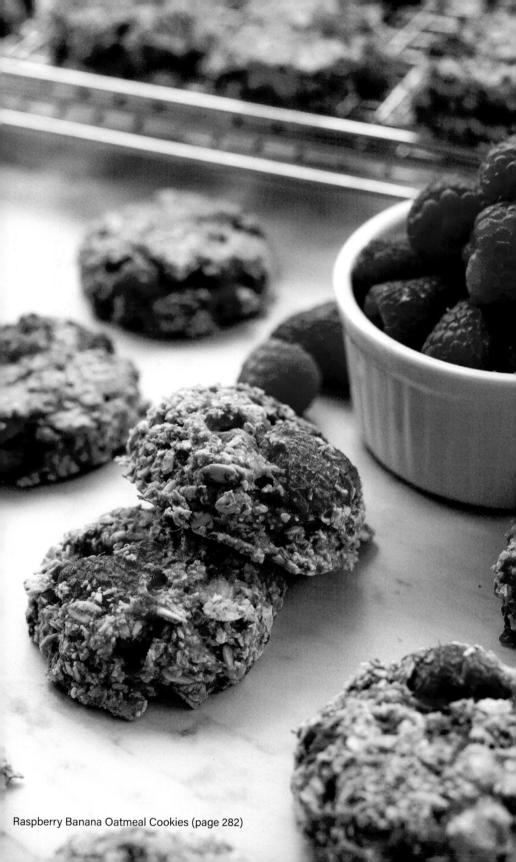

Raspberry Banana Oatmeal Cookies (page 282)

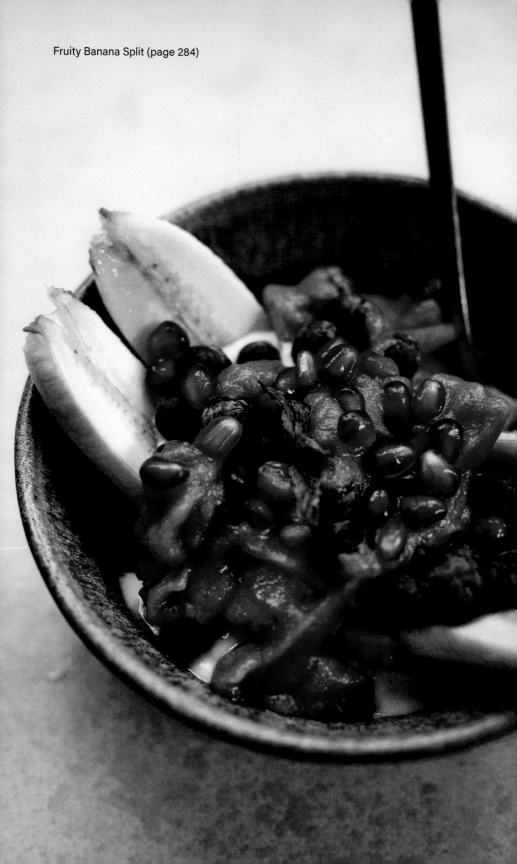

Fruity Banana Split (page 284)

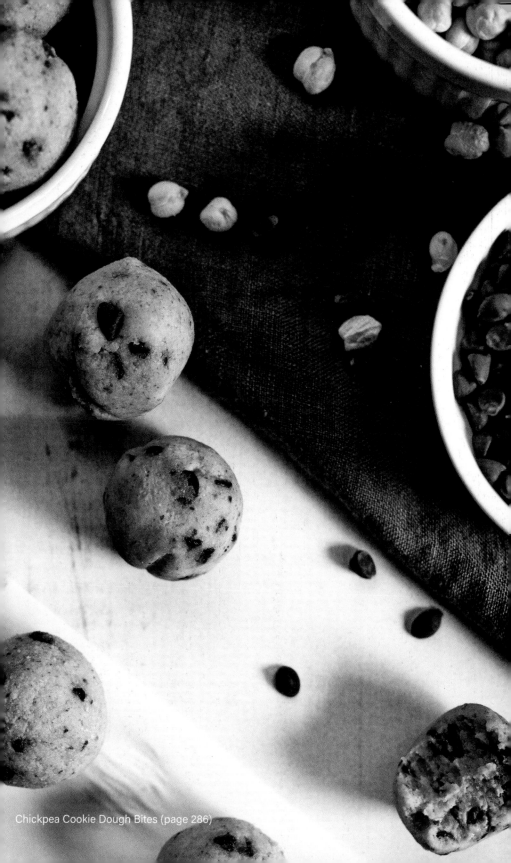

Chickpea Cookie Dough Bites (page 286)

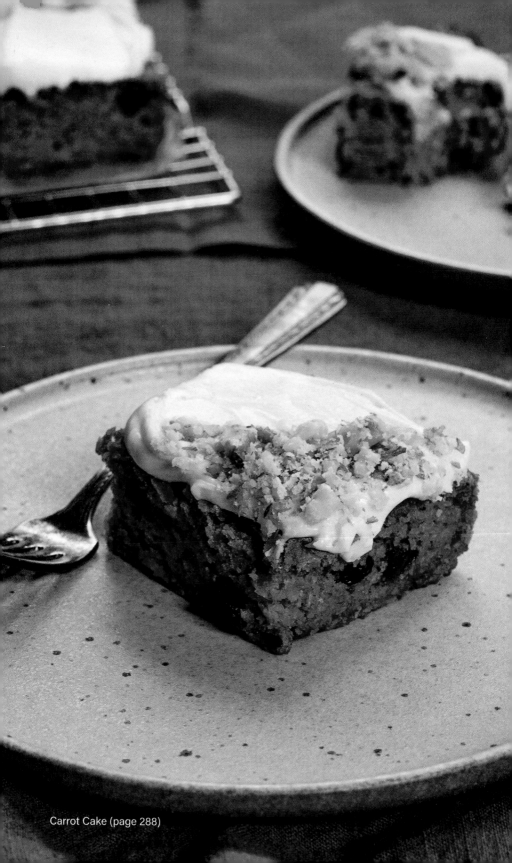

Carrot Cake (page 288)

Cheese and Broccoli Soup

SERVES 6   *Easy*

2 cups low-sodium vegetable broth

4 cups broccoli, cut into tiny florets (2–3 florets should fit on
   a spoonful)

6 cups (1 batch) Carrot Cauliflower Cheese Sauce (page 290)

Crushed red pepper (optional)

Add the broth to a stockpot and bring to a boil. Add the broccoli
florets and cover the pot; continue to boil for 3 to 4 minutes, until the
broccoli is fork-tender. Add the cheese sauce and mix until well combined. Let simmer for 4 minutes, or until the soup is heated through.

Divide among bowls and serve warm with a pinch of crushed red
pepper, if using.

PER SERVING (2 CUPS): 71 CALORIES, 5 G PROTEIN, 10 G CARBOHYDRATE,
1 G SUGAR, 0 G TOTAL FAT, 2% CALORIES FROM FAT, 1 G SATURATED FAT,
2 G FIBER, 260 MG SODIUM

—*DH*

Chickpea Pot Pie Stew with
Herbed Polenta Dumplings

SERVES 8   *Elegant*

FOR THE DUMPLINGS:

¾ cup whole-wheat flour

¾ cup stone-ground polenta

¼ cup nutritional yeast

1 tablespoon baking powder

1 teaspoon dried rosemary

1 teaspoon dried basil

½ teaspoon sea salt

1 cup unsweetened almond milk

¼ cup unsweetened applesauce

To make the dumplings, add the flour, polenta, nutritional yeast, baking powder, rosemary, basil, and salt to a bowl and whisk to combine. Add the milk and applesauce and mix with a spatula until a wet dough forms. Set aside.

FOR THE STEW:

1 onion, roughly chopped

2 carrots, thinly sliced

2 celery stalks, thinly sliced

2 tablespoons water or vegetable broth, plus more as needed

4 cloves garlic, minced

2 russet potatoes (skin on), diced small

1½ cups frozen peas

1½ cups frozen corn

1 (15.5-ounce) can low-sodium chickpeas, drained and
    rinsed, or 1½ cups cooked chickpeas

6 cups low-sodium vegetable broth

2 teaspoons poultry seasoning

1½ teaspoons sea salt

1 teaspoon black pepper

2 tablespoons cornstarch

½ cup water

Scallions or chives, thinly sliced, for garnish (optional)

Heat a large stockpot over medium heat. Add the onions, carrots, and celery and sauté 6 minutes, or until the onions are soft and translucent. Use 2 tablespoons of water or vegetable broth to prevent the vegetables from sticking to the pot; add more liquid as needed. Add the garlic and sauté 1 additional minute, or until fragrant, adding more liquid if needed.

Add the potatoes, peas, corn, chickpeas, broth, poultry seasoning, salt, and pepper to the pot; cover and bring the soup to a boil. Reduce to a simmer.

Add the cornstarch and water to a small bowl and whisk to combine and create a slurry. Stir the slurry into the stew until well combined.

Use a ¼-cup measuring spoon to scoop the dumpling dough onto the top of the stew; there should be 8 dumplings. Allow them to touch as they sit on top of the stew. Cover the pot and let the stew simmer and the dumplings cook for 20 to 22 minutes, until the tops of the dumplings are dry.

Divide the stew among bowls and top with dumplings; garnish with scallions or chives, if using.

PER SERVING (1¼ CUPS/1 DUMPLING): 243 CALORIES, 10 G PROTEIN, 48 G CARBOHYDRATE, 8 G SUGAR, 2 G TOTAL FAT, 3% CALORIES FROM FAT, 0 G SATURATED FAT, 9 G FIBER, 547 MG SODIUM

—DH

Speedy One-Pot Dal

SERVES 6   *Elegant*

---

1 onion, chopped

2 tablespoons vegetable broth or water, plus more as needed

5 cloves garlic, minced

1 tablespoon minced fresh ginger or ginger from a squeeze tube

1 (14.5-ounce) can diced tomatoes

1½ cups dried red lentils

¼ teaspoon crushed red pepper

4 cups low-sodium vegetable broth

¾ cup unsweetened almond milk

1 tablespoon garam masala

1 teaspoon turmeric

1 teaspoon sea salt

Juice of ½ lemon

Brown rice (optional)

Heat a saucepot over medium heat. Add the onion and sauté 6 minutes, or until translucent and soft; use 2 tablespoons vegetable broth or water to prevent the onion from sticking to the pot. Add the garlic and ginger and sauté 1 additional minute, or until fragrant, adding more liquid as needed.

Add the tomatoes, lentils, crushed red pepper, and vegetable broth and bring to a boil. Reduce to a simmer and let cook for 16 to 18 minutes, until the lentils are cooked through and soft. Add the milk, masala, turmeric, salt, and lemon juice and stir to combine. Let it cook over medium-low heat for 2 to 4 minutes to heat through.

Serve over brown rice, if desired.

PER SERVING (1 CUP): 222 CALORIES, 14 G PROTEIN, 38 G CARBOHYDRATE, 3 G SUGAR, 1 G TOTAL FAT, 1% CALORIES FROM FAT, 0 G SATURATED FAT, 15 G FIBER, 556 MG SODIUM

—DH

Mango Dal

SERVES 2 TO 4 | *Easy*

¼ cup vegetable broth

1 small onion, diced

2–4 cloves garlic, minced

1–3 teaspoons minced fresh ginger (optional)

1 tablespoon diced green chilies (optional)

½ teaspoon ground cumin

⅛ teaspoon turmeric, for color (optional)

1 cup red lentils or yellow split peas

1–3 teaspoons prepared yellow mustard

1–2 cups frozen mango cubes

3 cups water or vegetable broth

Salt

Cooked brown rice, for serving

Coconut flakes, for garnish (optional)

Lime, for garnish (optional)

Pour ¼ cup broth into a skillet. Sauté the onion, garlic, ginger, and green chilies, if using, until the onions are translucent. Stir in the cumin, turmeric, lentils, yellow mustard, and mango, plus 3 cups water or additional broth. Cover and bring to a boil. Reduce the heat to low and simmer, stirring occasionally, until the lentils or split peas are falling apart, 15 to 60 minutes (see note).

If the dal is too thick, thin with additional water or broth. Add salt to taste. Serve over cooked rice garnished with coconut flakes and a squeeze of fresh lime juice, if using (recommended).

Note: This recipe can also be prepared in a pressure cooker: Sauté, then pressure-cook 4 to 6 minutes; use natural release. Green chilies are sold diced or whole in a can, usually in the international or Mexican foods section of a supermarket. Red lentils take 15 to 20 minutes and yellow split peas take closer to 60 minutes.

PER SERVING (½ OF RECIPE, WITHOUT RICE): 411 CALORIES, 26 G PROTEIN, 75 G CARBOHYDRATE, 14 G SUGAR, 1 G TOTAL FAT, 2% CALORIES FROM FAT, 0.2 G SATURATED FAT, 32 G FIBER, 38 MG SODIUM

—*LN*

Orzo Chili

SERVES 4   *Easy*

1 quart low-sodium vegetable broth

1 small onion, diced

1–3 cloves garlic, minced

1–2 bell peppers (any colors), seeded and diced

1–2 tablespoons chili powder

1–3 teaspoons dried oregano

1 (28-ounce) can fire-roasted diced tomatoes

1 cup orzo or dry brown rice

1 (15-ounce) can low-sodium kidney beans or black beans,
    drained and rinsed

Salt and pepper

Hot sauce, for garnish (optional)

Pour ¼ cup of the broth into a large pot. Add the onions, garlic, and bell peppers. Sauté until the onions are translucent. Stir in the chili powder and oregano to coat.

Add 2 cups of the remaining broth, the tomatoes with juices, and orzo or rice. Stir together, cover, and bring to a boil. Reduce heat to low and simmer, stirring often, until the orzo is cooked, about 10 minutes (adjust time to 40 minutes for brown rice; do not stir).

Once the orzo is cooked, stir in the beans. Thin the chili with additional broth as desired. Season with salt and pepper. Garnish with a drizzle of hot sauce, if desired.

Note: For a stronger tomato flavor, add 1 to 4 tablespoons tomato paste. If you have the time, simmer on the stove for as long as possible or make ahead; the flavors only get better with time.

PER SERVING (¼ OF RECIPE): 348 CALORIES, 18 G PROTEIN, 63 G CARBO-HYDRATE, 13 G SUGAR, 3 G TOTAL FAT, 4% CALORIES FROM FAT, 1 G SATU-RATED FAT, 10 G FIBER, 54 MG SODIUM

—LN

Pasta e Fagioli

SERVES 4 *Easy*

½ cup small pasta (e.g., elbow macaroni, shells, or ditalini)

1 quart low-sodium vegetable broth

1 small yellow onion, diced

3–4 cloves garlic, minced

1 tablespoon Italian seasoning

¼ teaspoon dried basil

¼ teaspoon rubbed sage (optional)

1 (14-ounce) can fire-roasted diced tomatoes

1–2 celery stalks, diced

1–2 small carrots, diced

8 ounces green beans, trimmed and cut into 2-inch pieces

1 (15-ounce) can low-sodium kidney beans, cannellini beans, or lentils, drained and rinsed

Salt and pepper

Fresh basil or parsley, for garnish (optional)

Vegan Parmesan, for garnish (optional)

Cook the pasta al dente (see package for directions). Set the prepared pasta aside.

Pour ¼ cup of the broth into a large pot. Sauté the onions and garlic until the onions are translucent. Stir in the dried herbs to coat. Add the tomatoes with juices. Use your spatula to break up any large tomato pieces. Stir in the diced celery and carrots.

Continue to cook until just tender, adding broth as needed. Add 2 cups of the broth, green beans, and canned beans. Cover, bring to a boil, then reduce heat to low. Simmer for 5 to 20 minutes, until all vegetables reach the desired tenderness. Stir in the cooked pasta. Thin the soup with remaining broth as desired. Add salt and pepper to taste. If the soup is acidic, add a pinch of sugar. Stir in fresh basil or use as a garnish with vegan Parmesan, if desired.

Note: Tomato sauce or "tomatoes with Italian seasonings" can be substituted. For a stronger tomato broth flavor, stir in 1 to 3 table-spoons of tomato paste. Cooked brown rice, about 1 to 2 cups, can be substituted for the pasta. You may need to add additional broth to any soup leftovers.

PER SERVING (¼ OF RECIPE): 208 CALORIES, 14 G PROTEIN, 35 G CARBOHY-DRATE, 6 G SUGAR, 2 G TOTAL FAT, 3% CALORIES FROM FAT, 1 G SATURATED FAT, 9 G FIBER, 27 MG SODIUM

—LN

Mexican Noodle Soup

SERVES 4 *Easy*

4–6 cups vegetable broth

½ medium onion, diced

3–4 cloves garlic, minced

1 (14-ounce) can fire-roasted diced tomatoes

1 teaspoon dried oregano

½–1 teaspoon ground cumin

Light dash of paprika (optional)

Pinch of red pepper flakes (optional)

6 ounces noodles (e.g., spaghetti)

1 zucchini, diced (optional)

¼ cup frozen corn (optional)

1 (15-ounce) can pinto beans, drained and rinsed (optional)

Salt and pepper (optional)

Fresh cilantro (optional)

Corn tortilla chips (optional)

1 lime

Pour ¼ cup broth into a large pot. Sauté the onions and garlic until the onions are translucent. Transfer to a blender. Add the tomatoes with their juices and 1½ cups of the broth. Blend until smooth.

Transfer back to the pot. Add the oregano and cumin, plus paprika and pepper flakes, if using. Simmer for 1 to 2 minutes. Stir in 2 to 3 more cups of the broth and the noodles. Add the zucchini and corn as well, if using.

Cover and bring to a boil. Reduce the heat to low and simmer 7 to 15 minutes, until the noodles are cooked. Add beans, if using. Thin the soup with additional broth or water, if desired. Add salt and pepper to taste, if desired. Garnish with cilantro or corn chips, if desired. Cut the lime into quarters and serve with the soup. Squeeze lime juice over the top before eating.

Note: "Fire-roasted tomatoes with green chilies" can be substituted to make a spicer version. Hot sauce is a nice addition.

PER SERVING (¼ OF RECIPE): 226 CALORIES, 2 G PROTEIN, 44 G CARBOHY-DRATE, 2 G SUGAR, 2 G TOTAL FAT, 2% CALORIES FROM FAT, 0 G SATURATED FAT, 5 G FIBER, 56 MG SODIUM

—LN

Southwest Chili

SERVES 2 TO 4 *Easy*

2 cups low-sodium vegetable broth

1 small onion, diced

2 garlic cloves, minced

1 bell pepper (any color), diced

1 jalapeño, finely chopped, or minced green chilies (optional)

1–2 teaspoons ground cumin

1–2 tablespoons chili powder

1 (14-ounce) can diced tomatoes

2 (15-ounce) cans low-sodium black beans, drained and
    rinsed

1 cup frozen fire-roasted corn

½ teaspoon sugar (optional)

Salt and pepper

Pour ¼ cup of the broth into a large pot. Sauté the onions, garlic, and bell pepper, plus the jalapeño, if using, until the onions are translucent. Stir in the cumin and chili powder to coat. Cook 1 minute.

Add the tomatoes with juices, canned beans, corn, and all the remaining broth. Cover and bring to a boil. Reduce the heat to low and simmer for 5 to 15 minutes. If the chili is acidic, add the sugar.

Optional: Transfer 1 to 1½ cups chili to a blender and puree until smooth; stir back in. Add salt and pepper to taste plus additional broth, if desired.

Note: 2 cups salsa (traditional or salsa verde) may be substituted for the tomatoes, onions, and garlic. Quartered mushrooms can be added for a meaty bite. Sliced green onions, avocado, lime juice, cilantro, hot sauce, crumbled corn chips, vegan cheese, or vegan sour cream all make wonderful garnishes. Serve chili over cooked brown rice or a baked potato for a different meal.

PER SERVING (½ OF RECIPE): 354 CALORIES, 21 G PROTEIN, 64 G CARBO-HYDRATE, 14 G SUGAR, 4 G TOTAL FAT, 6% CALORIES FROM FAT, 1 G SATU-RATED FAT, 15 G FIBER, 204 MG SODIUM

—*LN*

Easy Quinoa and Broccoli Tabbouleh

SERVES 8 *Easy*

1½ cups cooked quinoa

1½ cups broccoli, chopped into tiny pieces

1 cup peeled and diced cucumber

1 cup halved cherry tomatoes

1 cup chopped fresh parsley

½ cup chopped fresh mint

¼ cup thinly sliced scallions

Juice of 1 lemon

½ teaspoon sea salt

½ teaspoon ground black pepper

Add the quinoa, broccoli, cucumber, tomatoes, parsley, mint, and scallions to a bowl. Mix to combine all of the ingredients. Add the lemon juice, salt, and pepper. Mix one more time to combine and coat everything with the wet ingredients.

PER SERVING (¾ CUP): 58 CALORIES, 2 G PROTEIN, 9 G CARBOHYDRATE, 1 G SUGAR, 1 G TOTAL FAT, 2% CALORIES FROM FAT, 0 G SATURATED FAT, 2 G FIBER, 154 MG SODIUM

—DH

Massaged Kale Caesar

SERVES 4   *Easy*

8 cups torn curly kale, stems removed

½ cup Creamy Caesar Dressing (page 291), plus more as
   desired

2 tablespoons nutritional yeast

1½ cups shredded carrots

1 cup halved cherry tomatoes

Oil-Free Crispy Chickpea Croutons (page 296—optional)

Freshly cracked black pepper (optional)

Add the kale to a large bowl. Drizzle with the caesar dressing and use your hands to massage the dressing into the pieces of kale. Add the nutritional yeast and the carrots and toss with the massaged kale to combine.

Divide among 4 bowls and top with cherry tomatoes. Add the chickpea croutons and pepper, if using.

PER SERVING (¼ OF RECIPE): 184 CALORIES, 8 G PROTEIN, 19 G CARBO-HYDRATE, 2 G SUGAR, 10 G TOTAL FAT, 5% CALORIES FROM FAT, 2 G SATU-RATED FAT, 4 G FIBER, 376 MG SODIUM

—*DH*

Pinto Picnic Salad

SERVES 4   *Easy*

4 cups baby spinach, roughly chopped

½ cup thinly sliced red onion

½ red bell pepper, thinly sliced

½ yellow bell pepper, thinly sliced

1 cup halved cherry tomatoes

1 cup peeled and diced papaya or mango

2 cups cooked brown rice, cooled completely

1 (15.5-ounce) can low-sodium pinto beans, drained and
     rinsed, or 1½ cups cooked pinto beans

Juice of 3 limes

2 tablespoons maple syrup

1 teaspoon chili powder

½ teaspoon smoked paprika

½ teaspoon salt

Add the spinach, onion, red pepper, yellow pepper, tomatoes, papaya, brown rice, and beans to a large container with a lid.

Add the lime juice, maple syrup, chili powder, smoked paprika, and salt to a small container with a lid and shake to combine.

When you reach your picnic destination, drizzle the dressing onto the salad in the big container. Place the lid on the big container and shake the contents to evenly disperse the dressing and coat everything.

Eat right out of the container or set out at the picnic for everyone to serve themselves.

PER SERVING (¼ OF RECIPE): 223 CALORIES, 10 G PROTEIN, 57 G CARBO-HYDRATE, 12 G SUGAR, 2 G TOTAL FAT, 3% CALORIES FROM FAT, 0 G SATU-RATED FAT, 10 G FIBER, 364 MG SODIUM

—*DH*

Rainbow Fajita Bowls

SERVES 2   *Easy*

½ red onion, thinly sliced

½ orange bell pepper, thinly sliced

1 large portobello cap, thinly sliced

½ cup fresh or frozen corn kernels

1 tablespoon low-sodium tamari

Juice of 2 limes

2 teaspoons reduced-sodium fajita or taco seasoning

4 cups roughly chopped romaine lettuce

1 cup roughly chopped purple cabbage

¼ cup halved cherry tomatoes

Brown rice (optional)

Pinto beans (optional)

Creamy Tofu Sauce (page 304), for garnish (optional)

Scallions, thinly sliced, for garnish (optional)

Add the onion, bell pepper, portobello, corn, tamari, lime juice, and fajita seasoning to a large bowl and toss to coat the vegetables with the liquid and seasoning.

Heat a large skillet over medium heat. Add the vegetable mixture and sauté for 6 minutes, until the onions are translucent and the mushrooms have decreased slightly in size, stirring frequently.

Add the romaine and cabbage to a bowl and toss to combine. Divide the romaine mixture among 2 bowls. Top with the tomatoes and fajita vegetables.

Add a scoop of rice and pinto beans, if using. Drizzle with the creamy tofu sauce, if using. Sprinkle with scallions, if using.

PER SERVING (½ OF RECIPE): 101 CALORIES, 4 G PROTEIN, 20 G CARBOHY-DRATE, 8 G SUGAR, 1 G TOTAL FAT, 1% CALORIES FROM FAT, 0 G SATURATED FAT, 5 G FIBER, 402 MG SODIUM

—*DH*

Loaded Choppy Salad Bowls

SERVES 4 *Elegant*

FOR THE DRESSING:

2 tablespoons tahini

Juice of 1 lemon

2 tablespoons tamari

2 tablespoons nutritional yeast flakes

1 tablespoon flax meal

2 teaspoons onion powder

1 teaspoon garlic powder

¼ cup water

FOR THE SALAD:

6 cups torn curly kale, stems removed

2 cups baby arugula

1 cup extra-firm tofu, drained and cut into ½-inch cubes

1 cup cooked chickpeas, drained

½ cup halved grape tomatoes

½ cup roughly chopped cucumber

½ cup shredded carrots

⅓ cup pitted green olives

1 apple (any variety), core removed and roughly chopped

¼ cup pomegranate seeds, for garnish (optional)

To make the dressing, add the tahini, lemon juice, tamari, nutritional yeast, flax meal, onion powder, garlic powder, and water to a bowl and whisk to combine.

To make the salad, add the kale, arugula, tofu, chickpeas, tomatoes, cucumber, carrots, olives, and apple to a large bowl and toss to combine all of the ingredients. If desired, set the mixed salad out on a large cutting board in batches to further chop everything to smaller pieces to create a chopped salad texture. Transfer back to the large bowl and drizzle with the dressing; toss to coat the salad.

Divide among 4 bowls and sprinkle each bowl with a tablespoon
of pomegranate seeds, if using.

PER SERVING (¼ OF RECIPE): 353 CALORIES, 24 G PROTEIN, 33 G CARBO-
HYDRATE, 4 G SUGAR, 14 G TOTAL FAT, 4% CALORIES FROM FAT, 2 G SATU-
RATED FAT, 11 G FIBER, 493 MG SODIUM

—DH

Roasted Maple Balsamic Brussels Sprouts and Sweet Potatoes

SERVES 8   *Easy*

2 medium sweet potatoes, peeled and cut into ½-inch cubes

3 cups brussels sprouts, trimmed and halved

1 teaspoon garlic powder

½ teaspoon sea salt

¼ teaspoon ground black pepper

2 tablespoons maple syrup

1 tablespoon balsamic vinegar

Fresh thyme leaves, for garnish (optional)

Preheat the oven to 425°F. Line a large baking sheet with parchment
paper.

Add the potatoes to the prepared baking sheet and bake for
15 minutes. Remove from the oven and add the brussels sprouts.
Sprinkle the potatoes and brussels sprouts with garlic powder, sea
salt, and black pepper. Drizzle with the maple syrup and toss with a
spatula to coat all pieces evenly.

Bake for an additional 15 minutes, or until the pieces of potato and
brussels sprouts are starting to brown and are fork-tender. Remove
from the oven, drizzle with the balsamic vinegar, and toss to coat.
Transfer to a serving dish and garnish with fresh thyme leaves, if using.

PER SERVING (ROUGHLY ¾ CUP): 100 CALORIES, 2 G PROTEIN, 17 G CAR-
BOHYDRATE, 6 G SUGAR, 4 G TOTAL FAT, 4% CALORIES FROM FAT, 1 G SATU-
RATED FAT, 3 G FIBER, 170 MG SODIUM

—DH

Chilled Pasta Primavera Salad

SERVES 8   *Easy*

8 ounces whole-wheat rotini pasta

2 cups broccoli florets, cut into small bite-sized pieces

½ small red onion, thinly sliced

½ red bell pepper, thinly sliced

½ cup watercress

1 cup thinly sliced yellow squash

1 cup thinly sliced zucchini

1 cup shredded carrots

2 tablespoons chopped fresh parsley

Juice of 1 lemon

2 tablespoons red wine vinegar

¼ cup nutritional yeast

1 tablespoon Italian seasoning

½ teaspoon sea salt

½ teaspoon ground black pepper

¼ teaspoon crushed red pepper

Cook the pasta according to package directions with enough water
to add the broccoli eventually. In the last 2 minutes of cooking, add
the broccoli and continue to cook for about 2 minutes, until the
pasta is al dente and the broccoli is easily pierced with a fork, but
not mushy. Drain the contents of the pot into a colander.

Transfer the pasta and broccoli to a large mixing bowl. Add the onion, red pepper, watercress, squash, zucchini, carrots, and parsley. Toss to combine.

Add the lemon juice and vinegar and toss to coat the ingredients. Add the nutritional yeast, Italian seasoning, salt, pepper, and crushed red pepper and toss to combine.

Let the salad chill for 30 minutes before serving, stirring occasionally to cool the ingredients all the way through.

PER SERVING (ROUGHLY 1 CUP): 144 CALORIES, 6 G PROTEIN, 27 G CARBO-HYDRATE, 3 G SUGAR, 1 G TOTAL FAT, 3% CALORIES FROM FAT, 0 G SATURATED FAT, 5 G FIBER, 175 MG SODIUM

—DH

Scalloped Potatoes

SERVES 8 *Elegant*

1 onion, thinly sliced

2 tablespoons vegetable broth or water, plus more as needed

4 cloves garlic, thinly sliced

1½ teaspoons dried rosemary

1 teaspoon sea salt

½ teaspoon black pepper

3 pounds Yukon gold potatoes, thinly sliced

4 cups Carrot Cauliflower Cheese Sauce (page 290)

Smoked paprika, for garnish (optional)

Chopped fresh parsley, for garnish (optional)

Preheat the oven to 400°F. Line a 9 x 13-inch baking dish with parchment paper.

Heat a large skillet over medium heat. Add the onions and sauté for 4 to 6 minutes, until translucent and soft; add 2 tablespoons vegetable broth or water to the skillet to prevent the onion from sticking or burning. Add the garlic, rosemary, salt, and pepper. Sauté for 2 more minutes, or until the garlic is fragrant, adding more liquid as needed.

Line the baking dish with half of the potatoes. Top the potatoes with the onion and garlic mixture, and 2 cups of the cheese sauce. Top with the remainder of the potatoes and cover with the remainder of the cheese sauce. Sprinkle with smoked paprika, if using. Bake for 60 minutes; it should be bubbly, and the edges will be starting to brown. Test the potato to make sure it is fork-tender. If it isn't tender yet, cook for an additional 10 to 15 minutes.

Remove from the oven and let cool for 10 minutes before serving. Sprinkle with parsley, if using.

PER SERVING (ROUGHLY 1 CUP): 214 CALORIES, 6 G PROTEIN, 30 G CARBO-HYDRATE, 2 G SUGAR, 8 G TOTAL FAT, 4% CALORIES FROM FAT, 1 G SATU-RATED FAT, 4 G FIBER, 179 MG SODIUM

—DH

Crispy Oil-Free Oven-Baked Potato Wedges

SERVES 2   *Convenient*

2 large russet potatoes, cut into wedges
1 tablespoon low-sodium tamari or soy sauce
1 teaspoon Italian seasoning
½ teaspoon sea salt
½ teaspoon ground black pepper
½ teaspoon garlic powder

Soak the potato wedges in a bowl of ice water for 20 minutes to remove the excess starch; this will allow them to crisp up nicely when baked.

Preheat the oven to 475°F. Line a baking sheet with parchment paper.

Drain the potatoes and toss with the tamari, Italian seasoning, salt, pepper, and garlic powder. Transfer to the prepared baking sheet, bake for 15 minutes, and flip the potatoes. Bake for an additional 15 minutes, or until crispy and golden brown.

PER SERVING (½ OF RECIPE): 122 CALORIES, 4 G PROTEIN, 28 G CARBOHY-DRATE, 1 G SUGAR, 0 G TOTAL FAT, 0% CALORIES FROM FAT, 0 G SATURATED FAT, 3 G FIBER, 584 MG SODIUM

—DH

Seaweed, Cucumber, and Chickpea Salad

SERVES 4   *Easy*

¼ cup rice vinegar

2 tablespoons tahini

2 tablespoons maple syrup

2 teaspoons low-sodium tamari or soy sauce

1 teaspoon white sesame seeds, plus more for garnish

3 Persian cucumbers, thinly sliced

1 (15.5-ounce) can low-sodium chickpeas, drained and rinsed, or 1½ cups cooked chickpeas

¼ cup wakame seaweed, soaked in warm water for 10 minutes and drained

Add the vinegar, tahini, maple syrup, tamari, and sesame seeds to a bowl and whisk to combine. Set aside.

Wrap the cucumbers in a paper towel and squeeze them dry over the sink. Add the cucumbers, chickpeas, wakame, and liquid mixture to a large bowl. Toss to combine.

Garnish with more sesame seeds, if desired.

PER SERVING (¼ OF RECIPE): 193 CALORIES, 7 G PROTEIN, 28 G CARBO-
HYDRATE, 10 G SUGAR, 6 G TOTAL FAT, 3% CALORIES FROM FAT, 1 G SATU-
RATED FAT, 5 G FIBER, 225 MG SODIUM

—DH

Twice-Baked Mediterranean Sweet Potatoes

SERVES 4   *Elegant*

4 large sweet potatoes
1 (15.5-ounce) can low-sodium chickpeas, drained and
    rinsed, or 1½ cups cooked chickpeas
1 Roma tomato, seeds removed and small-diced
¾ cup small-diced red onion
½ cup chopped roasted red pepper, drained from a jar
2 tablespoons roughly chopped capers
1 tablespoon finely chopped fresh dill or 1 teaspoon dried dill
1 teaspoon dried basil
¼ teaspoon sea salt
Juice of ½ lemon
White Bean Tzatziki (page 294—optional)
Chopped fresh parsley (optional)

Preheat the oven to 400°F. Line a baking sheet with parchment paper.

Pierce each potato with a fork several times and transfer to the
prepared baking sheet. Bake the potatoes for 50 to 60 minutes, until
a fork pierces through to the middle of the potato easily. Remove
from the oven and let rest until cool enough to handle.

Add the chickpeas, tomato, onion, red pepper, capers, dill, basil,
sea salt, and lemon juice to a bowl and mix to combine.

Cut one side off of each potato and scoop the insides out of each
one, leaving about ¼ inch of potato intact, being careful not to poke

holes in the skin. Transfer the insides of the potatoes to a large bowl and mash with a potato masher or fork. Add the chickpea mixture to the mashed sweet potatoes and stir to combine everything. Divide among the potato vessels; they will be overflowing.

Place the potatoes back in the oven and bake for 20 to 25 minutes, until heated through and the tops have started to brown.

Drizzle with tzatziki and sprinkle with parsley, if using.

PER SERVING (¼ OF RECIPE): 260 CALORIES, 8 G PROTEIN, 42 G CARBOHY-DRATE, 9 G SUGAR, 8 G TOTAL FAT, 3% CALORIES FROM FAT, 2 G SATURATED FAT, 9 G FIBER, 547 MG SODIUM

—DH

Rainbow Pad Thai Crunch Bowls

SERVES 6   *Easy*

FOR THE DRESSING:

¼ cup unsweetened natural peanut butter or almond butter

2 tablespoons water

2 tablespoons tamari or soy sauce

2 tablespoons rice vinegar

1 tablespoon maple syrup

Juice of 1 lime

2 teaspoons grated ginger or ginger from a squeeze tube

¼ teaspoon sea salt

FOR THE SALAD:

  2 cups torn curly kale, stems removed

  1 cup thinly sliced green cabbage

  1 cup thinly sliced red cabbage

  1 cup shredded carrot

  1 red bell pepper, thinly sliced

  1 cup thinly sliced sugar snap peas

  1 cup frozen edamame, cooked and cooled

  3 scallions, green and white parts, thinly sliced

  1 tablespoon chopped cilantro

  Crushed peanuts, for garnish (optional)

  Lime wedges, for garnish (optional)

In a bowl, whisk together the peanut butter, water, tamari, rice vinegar, maple syrup, lime juice, ginger, and sea salt. Set aside.

In a large bowl, combine the kale, green and red cabbage, carrot, bell pepper, peas, edamame, scallions, and cilantro. Toss to combine. Add the dressing and toss until everything is coated.

Garnish with crushed peanuts, if using. Serve with lime wedges to squeeze on individual servings, if desired.

Note: Use unsweetened sunflower butter if you want to avoid nut allergies.

PER SERVING (1½ CUPS): 86 CALORIES, 5 G PROTEIN, 13 G CARBOHYDRATE, 5 G SUGAR, 2 G TOTAL FAT, 3% CALORIES FROM FAT, 0 G SATURATED FAT, 3 G FIBER, 429 MG SODIUM

—DH

Creamy Broccoli Salad

SERVES 2 TO 4 *Convenient*

1 cup peas (optional)

3 cups broccoli florets

½ cup thick vegan yogurt (or vegan mayonnaise)

½–3 teaspoons pure maple syrup

1–2 tablespoons apple cider vinegar

Salt and pepper

Granulated garlic powder (optional)

Dijon mustard (optional)

1–4 tablespoons minced celery

1–4 tablespoons diced red onion

1–1½ cups halved seedless red grapes

1–4 tablespoons chopped walnuts

Microwave or thaw the peas as directed on the package, if using; set aside. Lightly steam the broccoli florets so they are bright green and al dente, but not soft, 2 to 4 minutes. Drain well and pat dry if necessary.

Refrigerate or place the broccoli in the freezer for a few minutes to cool down. Alternatively, leave the broccoli raw and chop it into very small pieces; set aside.

In a small bowl, whisk together the yogurt, ½ teaspoon maple syrup, and 1 tablespoon vinegar. Add more vinegar or maple syrup to taste, plus salt and pepper and/or garlic powder and/or Dijon mustard to taste, if using.

In a large bowl, toss together the prepared peas and broccoli, celery, and onion. Add the yogurt dressing and mix until well coated. Stir in the grapes and walnuts. For best results, chill for 5 to 15 minutes before serving.

Note: For best results, use a thicker vegan yogurt, not a thin or runny yogurt. For a lower fat version, replace walnuts with canned chickpeas or navy beans. Pecans may be substituted for walnuts.

PER SERVING (½ OF RECIPE): 260 CALORIES, 12 G PROTEIN, 32 G CAR-BOHYDRATE, 21 G SUGAR, 10 G TOTAL FAT, 13% CALORIES FROM FAT, 1 G SATURATED FAT, 6 G FIBER, 96 MG SODIUM

—LN

Creamy Coleslaw

SERVES 4   *Easy*

4 cups shredded cabbage
½ cup shredded carrot
3–4 tablespoons vegan mayonnaise
1–2 teaspoons apple cider vinegar
¼–½ teaspoon agave nectar
1 teaspoon Dijon mustard (optional)
¼–½ teaspoon celery seed, dill weed, or caraway seeds
   (optional)
Salt and pepper to taste

In a large bowl, toss together the cabbage and carrots; set aside. In a small bowl, whisk together the mayonnaise, 1 teaspoon vinegar, and a drop or two of agave nectar, plus the Dijon mustard and spices, if using. Add additional vinegar, agave nectar, and Dijon, plus salt and pepper to taste. Chill until serving.

Note: For simplicity, you can substitute half a bag (4 to 5 cups) of coleslaw mix or double the recipe to use up the entire bag. For a lower fat option, substitute a thick vegan yogurt (not a runny yogurt) or plain hummus. If using yogurt, you might want to add fresh lemon juice, about 1 to 1½ teaspoons. See page 302 for a low-fat mayo recipe.

PER SERVING (¼ OF RECIPE): 25 CALORIES, 1 G PROTEIN, 6 G CARBOHY-DRATE, 3 G SUGAR, 0 G TOTAL FAT, 0% CALORIES FROM FAT, 0 G SATURATED FAT, 2 G FIBER, 25 MG SODIUM

—*LN*

Riced Cauliflower Biryani

SERVES 2   *Easy*

¼ cup raisins

⅔ cup vegetable broth, divided

2–3 cloves garlic, minced

1 teaspoon minced fresh ginger root

½ small onion, diced

1–2 carrots, diced

¼–1 teaspoon ground cardamom

1 teaspoon garam masala

1 teaspoon ground turmeric

½ teaspoon mild yellow curry powder

½ teaspoon ground cumin

1 medium zucchini, diced

1 (16-ounce) bag frozen riced cauliflower

⅓ cup soy milk

Salt and pepper (optional)

Soak the raisins in boiling hot water for 10 minutes, or until plump. Discard the soaking water and set the raisins aside.

Pour ¼ cup of the broth into a skillet. Sauté the garlic, ginger, onions, and carrots until the onions are translucent. Stir in

¼ teaspoon cardamom, the garam masala, turmeric, curry powder, and cumin to coat. Cook for 1 minute. Add the zucchini, plus a splash of broth, if needed. Cook until the zucchini starts to soften, 1 to 3 minutes.

Stir in the riced cauliflower, soaked raisins, soy milk, and another ¼ cup of the broth. Cover and bring to a near boil. Reduce the heat to low and simmer for 10 minutes, or until most of the liquid has been absorbed and the carrots are tender.

Add 1 to 3 tablespoons additional broth (or soy milk) to moisten rice, if necessary or desired. Adjust spices to taste (e.g., add another ½ teaspoon garam masala or cardamon). Add salt and pepper to taste, if desired.

Note: For a full meal, add 1 (15-ounce) can lentils or chickpeas, drained and rinsed.

PER SERVING (½ OF RECIPE): 262 CALORIES, 10 G PROTEIN, 39 G CARBOHYDRATE, 22 G SUGAR, 11 G TOTAL FAT, 14% CALORIES FROM FAT, 9 G SATURATED FAT, 10 G FIBER, 375 MG SODIUM

—LN

Cornbread

SERVES 6   *Easy*

1 cup fine cornmeal

1 cup whole-wheat pastry flour

1 tablespoon baking powder

½ teaspoon salt

1 cup almond milk

¼ cup unsweetened applesauce

¼ cup maple syrup

Pinch of lemon zest (optional)

Preheat the oven to 400°F. Spritz a 9-inch glass pie dish with plant-based oil spray, if desired. In a mixing bowl, whisk together the cornmeal, flour, baking powder, and salt. In another bowl, whisk together the milk, applesauce, maple syrup, and zest, if using. Pour the wet mixture into the dry mixture. Stir to combine. Pour the batter into the prepared baking dish. Bake 20 minutes, or until firm in the center and golden.

Note: For a sweeter cornbread, add 2 or more tablespoons of raw sugar.

PER SERVING (⅙ OF RECIPE): 195 CALORIES, 4 G PROTEIN, 42 G CARBOHY-DRATE, 9 G SUGAR, 2 G TOTAL FAT, 2% CALORIES FROM FAT, 0 G SATURATED FAT, 4 G FIBER, 235 MG SODIUM

—LN

Green Bean Salad

SERVES 2   *Easy*

Balsamic-Dijon Vinaigrette (page 303) or store-bought
   balsamic dressing
1–4 tablespoons diced red onion
3 ounces pasta (any shape) or 1 (15-ounce) can chickpeas or
   navy beans, drained and rinsed
16 ounces fresh green beans, trimmed and cut into 1- to
   2-inch pieces
1 cup halved cherry tomatoes
1–3 tablespoons quartered Kalamata olives
Vegan feta cheese (optional)
Pine nuts (optional)
Salt and pepper (optional)

Prepare the balsamic-Dijon vinaigrette, if using, and set aside. Soak the diced red onion in cold water for 5 minutes; drain and set aside.

Cook the pasta as directed on the package but set a timer for half-way through the cooking time. At the halfway mark, add the green beans to the pot with the pasta.

Continue to cook until the pasta is tender, 4 to 5 more minutes. Drain and rinse thoroughly with cold water. Toss the pasta and green beans with about ¼ cup of the dressing. Gently fold in the tomatoes and olives, plus vegan feta and pine nuts, if using. Add another ¼ cup dressing or as much as you like. Season with salt and pepper, if desired. Serve immediately.

PER SERVING (½ OF RECIPE, WITHOUT DRESSING): 181 CALORIES, 8 G PRO-TEIN, 36 G CARBOHYDRATE, 4 G SUGAR, 2 G TOTAL FAT, 2% CALORIES FROM FAT, 0 G SATURATED FAT, 5 G FIBER, 31 MG CHOLESTEROL, 59 MG SODIUM

—LN

Potato Salad

SERVES 2   *Easy*

- 8 ounces red potatoes, cut into 1-inch pieces
- 2 tablespoons vegan mayonnaise (or hummus)
- 1½ teaspoons apple cider vinegar (or red wine vinegar)
- ½ teaspoon Dijon mustard
- 1–3 tablespoons minced celery
- 1–2 tablespoons fresh chives or diced red onion
- Salt and pepper (optional)

Place the potatoes into a medium pot. Cover the potatoes with cold water approximately 2 inches higher than the potatoes. Bring to a boil. Simmer until just tender, about 10 minutes. Drain, rinse with cold water, and drain again. Place the potatoes on a clean kitchen towel and gently pat them dry; set aside. In a large mixing bowl, stir together the mayonnaise, vinegar, and Dijon. Add the prepared potatoes, celery, and chives. Toss to gently coat. Add salt and pepper to taste, if desired. Add more mayonnaise, Dijon, or vinegar to taste, if desired.

Note: You can add chopped arugula (1 to 2 cups), parsley, minced dill pickle (or dill relish), smoked paprika, or Old Bay seasoning to make this your own. See page 302 for instructions on how to prepare low-fat vegan mayo.

PER SERVING (HALF OF RECIPE): 93 CALORIES, 3 G PROTEIN, 19 G CARBOHY-
DRATE, 2 G SUGAR, 0 G TOTAL FAT, 1% CALORIES FROM FAT, 0 G SATURATED
FAT, 2 G FIBER, 35 MG SODIUM

—LN

Asian-Inspired Rice Salad

SERVES 2   *Elegant*

Orange Ginger Dressing (page 305) or store-bought Asian-
    style dressing
½ cup frozen edamame
1½ cups cooked brown rice
2 clementine oranges, peeled and diced
1 green onion, sliced
1–2 cups shredded cabbage or coleslaw mix
Sliced almonds, for garnish (optional)
Sesame seeds, for garnish (optional)

Prepare the orange ginger dressing and set aside. Microwave or thaw the edamame as directed on the package. Toss the edamame, cooked rice, orange pieces, and green onion together.

Add the dressing and toss again. For best results, chill for an hour to allow flavors to blend. Garnish with almonds and sesame seeds before serving, if desired.

PER SERVING (½ OF RECIPE): 256 CALORIES, 8 G PROTEIN, 52 G CARBO-
HYDRATE, 10 G SUGAR, 3 G TOTAL FAT, 3% CALORIES FROM FAT, 0 G SATU-
RATED FAT, 6 G FIBER, 11 MG SODIUM

—*LN*

Cucumber Arame Salad

SERVES 4 *Easy*

1 cup arame (seaweed)
1 cup plus 2 tablespoons water
1 cucumber, peeled
½ teaspoon salt
2 tablespoons lemon juice
1 tablespoon rice vinegar
1 teaspoon low-sodium soy sauce
12 leaves butter lettuce

Soak the arame in 1 cup water for 15 minutes, or until it is soft.
Meanwhile, cut the cucumber lengthwise, scoop out the seeds, and
slice into thin crescents. Spread them on a plate, sprinkle with salt,
then put them in a bowl and let sit for 15 minutes. Drain thoroughly.

Drain the arame and add to the bowl of cucumber slices; stir in
the lemon juice, vinegar, soy sauce, and remaining water. Place 3 lettuce leaves on each plate and top with the arame-cucumber mixture.

PER SERVING (¼ OF RECIPE): 17 CALORIES, 2 G PROTEIN, 4 G CARBOHY-
DRATE, 1 G SUGAR, 0 G TOTAL FAT, 2% CALORIES FROM FAT, 2 G FIBER,
376 MG SODIUM

—*NB*

Perfect Brown Rice

SERVES 6 *Easy*

---

1 cup dry short-grain brown rice
3 cups water

Place the rice in a saucepan, rinse with water, then drain away the water. Place the pan on high heat and stir the rice until it is dry, about 2 minutes.

Add the 3 cups water. Bring to a boil, then simmer until the rice is thoroughly cooked but still retains just a hint of crunchiness—about 40 minutes. Drain off the remaining water. Do not cook the rice until all the water is absorbed. Top with soy sauce, sesame seeds, cooked vegetables, beans, or lentils, if desired.

PER ½-CUP SERVING (⅙ OF RECIPE): 115 CALORIES, 3 G PROTEIN, 24 G CAR-BOHYDRATE, 0 G SUGAR, 1 G FAT, 7% CALORIES FROM FAT, 0 G SATURATED FAT, 3 G FIBER, 5 MG SODIUM

—*NB*

Baked Falafel Bowls

SERVES 6	*Easy*

1 cup dry chickpeas, soaked in water overnight, drained and
   rinsed

½ cup roughly chopped red onion

½ cup parsley leaves

½ cup cilantro leaves

4 cloves garlic

½ teaspoon sea salt

½ teaspoon ground black pepper

½ teaspoon ground cumin

6 cups torn curly kale, stems removed

Red wine vinegar, to taste

1½ cups halved cherry tomatoes

1½ cups shredded carrots

¾ cup pitted kalamata olives

Easy Quinoa and Broccoli Tabbouleh (page 216—optional)

Classic Oil-Free Hummus (page 293—optional)

White Bean Tzatziki (page 294—optional)

Preheat the oven to 375°F. Line a baking sheet with parchment paper.

Add the chickpeas, onion, parsley, cilantro, garlic, salt, pepper, and cumin to a food processor and pulse the chickpeas into small crumbles. Pulse until everything is combined and a crumbly dough has formed.

Add the falafel dough to the prepared baking sheet, measuring out 1 level tablespoon for each falafel, and gently flatten into a disc. Bake for 15 minutes. Flip the falafel and bake for an additional 15 minutes. Turn the oven to broil and let broil for 3 to 5 minutes, until the tops are crispy. All broilers have different intensities, so be sure to keep an eye on your falafel so they don't burn.

Add the kale to a large bowl and drizzle it with red wine vinegar; use your hands to massage the vinegar into the kale. This will help break the kale down to make it easier to chew. Divide the kale among 6 bowls with tomatoes, carrots, olives, and falafel. Add tabbouleh and hummus, if using. Drizzle with white bean tzatziki, if using.

PER SERVING (⅙ OF RECIPE): 171 CALORIES, 9 G PROTEIN, 32 G CARBO-HYDRATE, 10 G SUGAR, 3 G TOTAL FAT, 2% CALORIES FROM FAT, 0 G SATU-RATED FAT, 6 G FIBER, 432 MG SODIUM

—DH

Easy Breezy Veggie Curry

SERVES 8 *Elegant*

2 cups peeled and roughly chopped carrots

3½ cups low-sodium vegetable broth, divided

1 tablespoon curry powder

½ teaspoon sea salt

1 onion, chopped

2 tablespoons water or vegetable broth

4 cloves garlic, minced

2 teaspoons minced fresh ginger or ginger from a squeeze tube

1 large russet potato, peeled and cut into ½-inch cubes

2 cups cauliflower florets, cut into bite-sized pieces

2 cups broccoli florets, cut into bite-sized pieces

1 (14.5-ounce) can diced tomatoes

1 (15.5-ounce) can low-sodium chickpeas

1 cup frozen peas

5 ounces baby spinach

Chopped fresh cilantro (optional)

Cooked brown rice (optional)

Add the carrots and 2 cups of the broth to a saucepot and bring to a boil. Reduce the heat and let simmer for 6 to 8 minutes, until the carrots are fork-tender. Transfer to a blender, add the curry powder and salt, and blend until smooth and creamy.

Heat a large nonstick skillet over medium heat. Add the onion and sauté for 4 minutes, or until the onion is translucent. Add 2 tablespoons of water or vegetable broth as needed to prevent the onion from sticking to the skillet. Add the garlic and ginger and sauté 1 additional minute, or until fragrant.

Add the potatoes and the remaining 1½ cups of broth, cover and bring to a boil, reduce to a simmer, and let cook for 4 minutes. Add the cauliflower, stir to combine, cover, and cook another 4 minutes, or until the potatoes are fork-tender.

Add the broccoli, tomatoes, chickpeas, peas, and carrot mixture; mix to combine everything and let it cook for 4 to 6 minutes, until the broccoli is tender and everything is heated through. Add the spinach and stir until the spinach is wilted and mixed in with everything. Season with more curry powder and salt to taste.

Serve hot, garnished with cilantro over brown rice, if using.

PER SERVING (1 CUP): 143 CALORIES, 8 G PROTEIN, 28 G CARBOHYDRATE, 5 G SUGAR, 1 G TOTAL FAT, 2% CALORIES FROM FAT, 0 G SATURATED FAT, 6 G FIBER, 497 MG SODIUM

—*DH*

Cauliflower and Chickpea Masala

SERVES 8   *Elegant*

1 onion, diced

2 cups cauliflower florets, cut into bite-sized pieces

2 tablespoons vegetable broth, plus more as needed

3 cloves garlic, minced

1 (15.5-ounce) can low-sodium chickpeas, drained and
   rinsed, or 1½ cups cooked chickpeas

1 (14.5-ounce) can diced tomatoes, with juices

2 tablespoons tomato paste

½ teaspoon sea salt

1 teaspoon ground ginger

1 teaspoon cumin powder

2 teaspoons garam masala

1 cup unsweetened almond milk

¼ teaspoon coconut extract (optional)

Brown rice (optional)

Chopped cilantro (optional)

Heat a large nonstick skillet over medium heat. Add the onion and cauliflower and sauté 6 minutes, or until the onions are soft. Add 2 tablespoons of vegetable broth to prevent the vegetables from sticking; add more liquid as needed. Add the garlic and sauté 1 additional minute, or until fragrant, adding more liquid as needed.

Add the chickpeas, diced tomatoes, tomato paste, salt, ginger, cumin, and masala and mix until well combined.

Add the milk, and coconut extract, if using; mix until well combined. Cover and bring to a simmer for 12 minutes, or until heated through, the cauliflower is tender, and the flavors have blended together.

Serve over rice sprinkled with fresh chopped cilantro, if desired.

PER SERVING (1 CUP): 81 CALORIES, 3 G PROTEIN, 11 G CARBOHYDRATE, 2 G SUGAR, 2 G TOTAL FAT, 3% CALORIES FROM FAT, 0 G SATURATED FAT, 4 G FIBER, 269 MG SODIUM

—DH

Baked Polenta with Mushroom Ragu

SERVES 8	*Elegant*

FOR THE POLENTA:

   3 cups low-sodium vegetable broth

   1 teaspoon sea salt

   1 cup stone-ground polenta

   ¼ cup nutritional yeast

Preheat the oven to 400°F. Line an 8 x 8-inch baking dish with parchment paper.

To make the polenta, add the broth and salt to a saucepot and bring to a boil. Slowly add the polenta and nutritional yeast while whisking to combine the ingredients. Lower to a simmer and stir frequently for 8 to 10 minutes, until the polenta has become very thick, almost firming up.

Transfer the mixture to the prepared baking dish and bake for 20 to 22 minutes, until golden brown on top. Remove from the oven and let cool slightly, then cut into 9 squares.

FOR THE MUSHROOM RAGU:

1 onion, chopped

1 (5-ounce) package sliced shiitake mushrooms

1 (8-ounce) package sliced baby bella or cremini mushrooms

2 tablespoons plus 1 cup vegetable broth, and more as
    needed

4 cloves garlic

½ teaspoon dried thyme

½ teaspoon dried oregano

½ teaspoon sea salt

¼ teaspoon ground black pepper

1 cup crushed tomatoes

2 tablespoons cornstarch

2 tablespoons chopped fresh parsley, plus more for garnish

1 tablespoon red wine vinegar

2 cups chopped kale

Creamy Tofu Sauce (page 304), for garnish (optional)

Heat a large nonstick skillet over medium heat. Add the onion, shiitake mushrooms, and baby bella mushrooms and sauté for 6 minutes, or until the onions are translucent and the mushrooms have reduced in size. Add 2 tablespoons of the vegetable broth to prevent vegetables from sticking; add more liquid as needed. Add the garlic and sauté 1 additional minute, or until fragrant, adding more liquid if needed.

Add the thyme, oregano, salt, and pepper and stir to combine. Add the crushed tomatoes and let simmer for 3 minutes to heat through.

Add 1 cup of the broth and the cornstarch to a small bowl and whisk to create a slurry. Add the slurry, the 2 tablespoons parsley, vinegar, and kale to the skillet and stir to combine. Let simmer for 2 to 4 minutes, until the kale has wilted and the mixture has thickened, then remove from heat.

To serve, add 1 piece of polenta to a plate and top with a scoop of mushroom ragu. Drizzle with creamy tofu sauce, if using. Sprinkle with the remaining parsley, if desired.

You will have one extra piece of polenta.

Note: This is a great recipe to make as dinner and use the leftover portions for meal prep for the rest of the week.

PER SERVING (⅛ OF RECIPE): 89 CALORIES, 6 G PROTEIN, 15 G CARBOHYDRATE, 4 G SUGAR, 0 G TOTAL FAT, 2% CALORIES FROM FAT, 0 G SATURATED FAT, 4 G FIBER, 580 MG SODIUM

—*DH*

Pesto Spaghetti with Broccoli and Sun-Dried Tomatoes

SERVES 6   *Elegant*

---

8 ounces whole-wheat or chickpea spaghetti

4 cups broccoli florets, cut into bite-sized pieces

1 cup julienned sun-dried tomatoes, not packed in oil

1 cup (1 batch) Power Greens Pesto (page 292)

Cook the pasta according to the package directions. Add the broccoli and sun-dried tomatoes to the pot the last 2 minutes of cooking. Reserve ¼ cup of the cooking water. Drain everything in a colander and transfer back to the pot.

Add the pesto and toss to combine. Add reserved cooking water if needed to evenly disperse the pesto. Serve hot.

PER SERVING (1½ CUPS): 125 CALORIES, 5 G PROTEIN, 18 G CARBOHY-
DRATE, 2 G SUGAR, 3 G TOTAL FAT, 3% CALORIES FROM FAT, 1 G SATURATED
FAT, 3 G FIBER, 23 MG SODIUM

—DH

One-Pot Cauliflower Piccata Pasta

SERVES 6   *Elegant*

1 onion, diced

1 head (roughly 4 cups) cauliflower, cut into bite-sized florets

2 tablespoons water or vegetable broth, plus more as needed

4 cloves garlic

8 ounces chickpea or whole-wheat rotini pasta

3 cups low-sodium vegetable broth, divided

1 tablespoon cornstarch

¼ cup capers

¼ cup chopped fresh parsley, plus more for garnish (optional)

Juice of 2 lemons

¼ teaspoon sea salt

¼ teaspoon ground black pepper

Crushed red pepper (optional)

Heat a large skillet with a lid over medium-high heat until the skillet is
very hot. Add the onions and cauliflower and sauté 4 minutes, or until
the onions are soft and translucent. Add 2 tablespoons of water or vegetable broth as needed to prevent sticking. Add the garlic and continue
to cook for 5 minutes, stirring frequently and adding liquid as needed.
The cauliflower may start to brown on the edges; that's okay.

Add the pasta and 2½ cups of the vegetable broth. Bring to a boil
and reduce to a simmer; cook for 8 minutes, stirring occasionally,
until the liquid has decreased by half and the pasta is al dente.

In a small bowl, combine the remaining ½ cup vegetable broth and the cornstarch; whisk to combine and create a slurry.

Add the capers, parsley, lemon juice, salt, and pepper to the pot; stir to combine. Add the slurry and stir to combine. Remove from the heat and let sit for 4 minutes to let the sauce thicken.

Serve hot, garnished with more parsley and crushed red pepper, if desired.

PER SERVING (1¼ CUPS): 88 CALORIES, 4 G PROTEIN, 17 G CARBOHYDRATE, 4 G SUGAR, 1 G TOTAL FAT, 2% CALORIES FROM FAT, 0 G SATURATED FAT, 4 G FIBER, 327 MG SODIUM

—DH

Chimichurri Chickpea Pasta

SERVES 6 *Easy*

8 ounces whole-wheat rotini pasta

1 (15.5-ounce) can low-sodium chickpeas, drained and
    rinsed, or 1½ cups cooked chickpeas

1 bunch asparagus, cut into 2-inch pieces

1 red bell pepper, thinly sliced

1 cup (1 batch) Chimichurri Sauce (page 295)

Chopped fresh parsley (optional)

Cook the pasta according to the package directions. Add the chickpeas, asparagus, and bell pepper to the pasta during the last 2 minutes of cooking. Reserve ½ cup cooking water; set aside. Drain the pasta mixture in a colander and transfer back to the pot.

Add the chimichurri sauce and mix to coat the vegetables and the pasta. Add some pasta water, as needed, to help evenly disperse the sauce.

Serve garnished with chopped fresh parsley, if using.

PER SERVING (1¼ CUPS): 282 CALORIES, 7 G PROTEIN, 17 G CARBOHYDRATE, 2 G SUGAR, 17 G TOTAL FAT, 6% CALORIES FROM FAT, 1 G SATURATED FAT, 5 G FIBER, 338 MG SODIUM

—DH

Sheet Pan Broccoli and Tofu Teriyaki

SERVES 6 *Easy*

FOR THE TOFU AND BROCCOLI:

1 (8-ounce) package cremini mushrooms, sliced

3 tablespoons low-sodium tamari or soy sauce, divided

1 (14-ounce) package extra-firm tofu, drained, patted dry, and cut into ½-inch cubes

1 tablespoon cornstarch

4 cups broccoli florets, cut into uniform pieces

Brown rice (optional)

Thinly sliced scallions, for garnish (optional)

White sesame seeds, for garnish (optional)

FOR THE TERIYAKI SAUCE:

⅓ cup low-sodium tamari or soy sauce

3 tablespoons water

2 tablespoons maple syrup

2 tablespoons rice vinegar or white vinegar

2 teaspoons grated fresh ginger or ginger from a squeeze tube

1 clove garlic, minced

1 teaspoon cornstarch

Preheat the oven to 425°F. Line a baking sheet with parchment paper.

To make the tofu and broccoli, add the mushrooms to a large bowl with 1 tablespoon of tamari; toss to coat. Transfer to the prepared baking sheet. Add the tofu to the same large bowl with

1 tablespoon of the remaining tamari and toss to coat. Sprinkle with the cornstarch and toss to coat. Add the tofu to the baking sheet and bake for 10 minutes. While the tofu and mushrooms are baking, add the broccoli to the same bowl and toss with the remaining 1 tablespoon of tamari.

Remove the tofu and mushrooms from the oven. Add the broccoli to the sheet pan and toss everything with a spatula to combine. Bake for an additional 15 minutes, or until the tofu is crispy and the broccoli is fork-tender.

For the teriyaki sauce, add the tamari, water, maple syrup, vinegar, ginger, garlic, and cornstarch to a small saucepot. Whisk everything to combine and dissolve the starch into the liquid. Heat over medium heat and bring to a simmer. Simmer for about 3 minutes, until the sauce thickens; it should coat the back of a spoon.

Add the tofu, broccoli, and mushrooms to a large bowl and toss with the teriyaki sauce. Serve over rice and garnish with scallions, and sesame seeds, if using.

PER SERVING (⅙ OF RECIPE): 129 CALORIES, 11 G PROTEIN, 13 G CARBOHY-DRATE, 5 G SUGAR, 3 G TOTAL FAT, 3% CALORIES FROM FAT, 1 G SATURATED FAT, 3 G FIBER, 535 MG SODIUM

—*DH*

Chilled Bok Choy Soba Noodle Bowls

SERVES 6 *Elegant*

¼ cup low-sodium tamari or soy sauce

¼ cup tahini

¼ cup water

2 tablespoons rice vinegar or white vinegar

2 tablespoons maple syrup

1 tablespoon black sesame seeds, plus more for garnish

1 cup shelled frozen edamame, thawed

1 cup snow peas or sugar snap peas, thinly sliced

½ cup shredded carrot

1 (14-ounce) package extra-firm tofu, drained and cut into
    ½-inch cubes

2 tablespoons water or vegetable broth

2 baby bok choy, sliced vertically into quarters

2 cups torn curly kale, stems removed

6 scallions with white part, thinly sliced

2 cups cooked soba noodles

Add the tamari, tahini, water, vinegar, maple syrup, and black sesame seeds to a bowl and whisk to combine; set aside.

Heat a large nonstick skillet over medium heat. Add the edamame, snow peas, carrots, and tofu to the skillet and sauté for 4 minutes; add 2 tablespoons of water or vegetable broth as needed to prevent sticking.

Add the bok choy, cover with a lid, and cook for an additional 4 to 6 minutes, until the bok choy is tender but still vibrant, and the liquid from the tofu has evaporated from the skillet. Add the kale and scallions and mix continuously for 1 to 2 minutes, until the kale has wilted and everything is well combined. Transfer the mixture to a large bowl.

Add the soba noodles to the bowl with the liquid mixture and toss everything to combine. Let chill in the refrigerator for 30 minutes before serving.

Serve garnished with more sesame seeds, if desired.

PER SERVING (2 CUPS): 270 CALORIES, 20 G PROTEIN, 25 G CARBOHYDRATE, 6 G SUGAR, 11 G TOTAL FAT, 4% CALORIES FROM FAT, 1 G SATURATED FAT, 4 G FIBER, 457 MG SODIUM

—DH

Egg Roll in a Bowl

SERVES 6   *Easy*

¼ cup low-sodium tamari or soy sauce

2 tablespoons tahini

2 tablespoons water, plus more as needed

1 tablespoon rice vinegar or white vinegar

1 tablespoon maple syrup

1 teaspoon fresh grated ginger or ginger from a squeeze tube

2 cloves garlic, minced

1 (14-ounce) package extra-firm tofu, drained

2 tablespoons nutritional yeast

½ teaspoon kala namak or sea salt

¼ teaspoon turmeric powder

1 (1-pound) bag tricolor coleslaw mix

Thinly sliced scallions, for garnish (optional)

Sriracha (optional)

Add the tamari, tahini, water, vinegar, maple syrup, ginger, and garlic to a bowl and whisk to combine. Set aside.

Heat a large nonstick skillet over medium heat. Crumble the tofu into the skillet, add the nutritional yeast, kala namak, and turmeric and toss to coat the tofu. If the tofu sticks, use 2 tablespoons of water to release the tofu.

Add the coleslaw mixture to the skillet and toss to combine. Add the liquid mixture and stir to coat all of the ingredients; let cook for 4 minutes, or until the cabbage has cooked down and reduced in size.

Serve garnished with scallions and drizzled with sriracha, if using.

PER SERVING (⅙ OF RECIPE): 152 CALORIES, 10 G PROTEIN, 13 G CARBOHY-DRATE, 5 G SUGAR, 6 G TOTAL FAT, 4% CALORIES FROM FAT, 1 G SATURATED FAT, 5 G FIBER, 514 MG SODIUM

—DH

Red Pepper and Artichoke Paella

SERVES 6   *Easy*

1 onion, chopped

1 red bell pepper, seeds removed and sliced

1 cup canned artichokes, drained, rinsed, and quartered

Water or vegetable broth

3 cloves garlic, minced

2 Roma tomatoes, diced

1 cup frozen peas, thawed

2 teaspoons paprika

1 teaspoon ground turmeric

1 teaspoon sea salt

2 cups cooked brown rice

Juice of 1 lemon

Chopped fresh parsley, for garnish (optional)

Heat a large nonstick skillet over medium-high heat. Add the onion, bell pepper, and artichokes and sauté for 6 minutes, or until soft. Add water or vegetable broth, 2 tablespoons at a time, as needed to prevent the vegetables from burning or sticking to the pan. Add the garlic and sauté for 1 additional minute, or until fragrant, adding more liquid as needed.

Add the tomatoes, peas, paprika, turmeric, and salt. Cook for 2 minutes, or until heated through.

Add the rice and lemon juice, mix well to combine, and cook an additional 2 minutes, or until heated through.

Serve hot, garnished with parsley, if desired.

PER SERVING (1¼ CUPS): 88 CALORIES, 5 G PROTEIN, 25 G CARBOHYDRATE, 5 G SUGAR, 1 G TOTAL FAT, 2% CALORIES FROM FAT, 0 G SATURATED FAT, 5 G FIBER, 461 MG SODIUM

—DH

Penne Arrabbiata

SERVES 4	*Elegant*

8 ounces whole-wheat penne pasta
1 batch Easy Arrabbiata Sauce (page 298)
Fresh basil leaves, for garnish (optional)
Vegan Parmesan, for garnish (optional)

Cook the pasta according to the package directions. Add the arrabbiata sauce to the hot cooked pasta and stir to combine until all the pasta is coated.

Serve hot, garnished with fresh basil leaves and Parmesan, if using.

Note: Add sautéed or steamed vegetables to make a heartier and more nutrient-packed pasta.

PER SERVING (¼ OF RECIPE): 313 CALORIES, 10 G PROTEIN, 49 G CARBOHY-DRATE, 9 G SUGAR, 8 G TOTAL FAT, 3% CALORIES FROM FAT, 0 G SATURATED FAT, 0 G FIBER, 462 MG SODIUM

—DH

Cheesy Broccoli Casserole

SERVES 2 TO 4   *Easy*

1 cup soy milk

⅓ cup nutritional yeast

2 tablespoons tomato paste or ketchup

1 tablespoon cornstarch

½ teaspoon granulated onion powder

½ teaspoon granulated garlic powder

½ cup canned pumpkin or canned butternut squash

8 ounces macaroni

2–4 cups frozen broccoli florets

1 (15-ounce) can vegan chili

In a saucepan, whisk together the soy milk, nutritional yeast, tomato paste, cornstarch, spices, and pumpkin until well combined. Heat over low heat until warm; set aside.

In another pot, cook the pasta as directed on the package, adding broccoli a minute or two before the pasta is done cooking. Drain. Stir the pasta and broccoli together with the prepared sauce. Stir in the vegan chili. Serve immediately.

PER SERVING (¼ OF RECIPE): 413 CALORIES, 22 G PROTEIN, 77 G CARBO-HYDRATE, 8 G SUGAR, 3 G TOTAL FAT, 4% CALORIES FROM FAT, 12 G FIBER, 68 MG SODIUM

—*LN*

Firecracker Bowls

SERVES 2 TO 3   *Convenient*

Tahini Dipping Sauce (page 305) or ¼ cup tahini

4–6 cups broccoli florets or kale or green beans

2 small sweet potatoes

1 (15-ounce) can chickpeas, drained

¼–½ cup sriracha

1–2 tablespoons agave nectar or maple syrup

Sesame seeds, for garnish (optional)

1–2 green onions, sliced, for garnish (optional)

Prepare the tahini dipping sauce, if using, and set aside. Steam or pressure-cook the broccoli, kale, or green beans to the desired tenderness and set aside. Microwave, bake, steam, or pressure-cook the sweet potatoes and set aside.

In a skillet, combine the chickpeas with the sriracha and agave nectar. Marinate for 5 or more minutes. Cook over medium-high heat, stirring, until caramelized. Alternatively, transfer the marinated chickpeas to a baking sheet lined with parchment paper and bake 25 to 45 minutes at 350°F, turning every 10 minutes, until crisp.

Slice the cooked sweet potatoes in half or cube or mash. Serve the prepared chickpeas and broccoli on top of the prepared sweet potatoes. Drizzle with the prepared tahini dipping sauce or tahini. Garnish with sesame seeds and green onions, if desired.

Note: For a lower fat version, whisk 1 to 4 teaspoons of nondairy milk into plain hummus to make a cream sauce for drizzling instead of tahini. Cubed tofu can replace chickpeas.

PER SERVING (½ OF RECIPE): 495 CALORIES, 16 G PROTEIN, 72 G CARBO-
HYDRATE, 16 G SUGAR, 18 G TOTAL FAT, 23% CALORIES FROM FAT, 2 G
SATURATED FAT, 13 G FIBER, 350 MG SODIUM

—*LN*

Lasagna Rolls

SERVES 4 *Elegant*

8 dry lasagna noodles
1 (24-ounce) jar vegan low-sodium marinara sauce
1 (10-ounce) package frozen spinach
1 (14-ounce) package firm tofu, drained and crumbled
1 teaspoon fresh lemon juice
¼ cup nutritional yeast
2 tablespoons Italian seasoning
¼ teaspoon granulated garlic powder
Salt and pepper (optional)
¼ cup vegan Parmesan or vegan mozzarella shreds, for garnish

Cook the lasagna noodles as directed on the package; drain and
rinse under cold water. Set aside.

Pour ½ cup of the marinara sauce into a large pot and spread it
around evenly; set aside. Microwave or cook the spinach as directed
on the package, then place in a colander. Use a spatula or the back of
a measuring cup to squeeze out any excess water and set the cooked
spinach aside.

Pat the prepared noodles dry and lay them flat on a cutting board.

Stir together the crumbled tofu, lemon juice, nutritional yeast,
Italian seasoning, garlic powder, and ¼ cup of the marinara sauce.
Stir the prepared spinach into the tofu mixture well. Add salt and
pepper, plus more garlic powder or Italian seasoning, to taste. Spread
½ cup of the tofu-spinach mixture onto each noodle. Roll up each

noodle and place it seam side down in the pot. Repeat this process with the remaining lasagna noodles.

Pour 2 to 3 cups of the marinara sauce over the prepared rolls. Cover and heat on low until warm. Using tongs, carefully transfer the lasagna rolls to a serving plate. Spoon marinara from the pot over the rolls. Garnish with vegan Parmesan and serve immediately.

PER SERVING (¼ OF RECIPE; 2 ROLLS): 570 CALORIES, 28 G PROTEIN, 86 G CARBOHYDRATE, 19 G SUGAR, 15 G TOTAL FAT, 19% CALORIES FROM FAT, 2 G SATURATED FAT, 11 G FIBER, 123 MG SODIUM

—LN

Personal Pita Pizza

SERVES 1   *Convenient*

TRADITIONAL:

    1 tablespoon warm water
    1–2 tablespoons tomato paste
    Dash of Italian seasoning
    Dash of dried basil
    Salt and pepper (optional)
    1 whole-wheat pita bread
    Pizza toppings (e.g., sliced black olives, broccoli, artichoke
        hearts, vegan cheese)

Preheat the oven or toaster oven to 425°F. In a small mixing bowl, whisk 1 tablespoon warm water into the tomato paste. Add a little more water if needed to make it spreadable. It should be thick, like hummus or creamy peanut butter. Add the Italian seasoning and dried basil to taste, plus salt and pepper, if desired. Don't be shy with the dried basil! Spread the "tomato sauce" out on the pita in a thin, even layer. Add the desired toppings. Bake 4 to 7 minutes, or until warm and the pita is lightly toasted but not burned or hard.

PER SERVING (ENTIRE RECIPE, EXCLUDING TOPPINGS): 184 CALORIES, 7 G PROTEIN, 38 G CARBOHYDRATE, 3 G SUGAR, 2 G TOTAL FAT, 2% CALORIES FROM FAT, 0 G SATURATED FAT, 5 G FIBER, 356 MG SODIUM

TROPICAL:

1–3 tablespoons Barbecue Sauce (page 301) or commercial brand barbecue sauce

1 whole-wheat pita bread

1–2 tablespoons diced pineapple

1–4 tablespoons canned black beans, rinsed and drained

Red onion or green onion, sliced (optional)

Cilantro (optional)

Preheat the oven or toaster oven to 425°F. Prepare the barbecue sauce recipe, if using. Spread a thin, even layer of barbecue sauce on the pita, about 3 to 4 tablespoons. Sprinkle the pineapple and black beans evenly on top. Bake for 4 to 7 minutes, until warm and the pita is lightly toasted but not burned or hard. Garnish with onion and cilantro, if using.

PER SERVING (ENTIRE RECIPE): 292 CALORIES, 9 G PROTEIN, 62 G CARBO-HYDRATE, 14 G SUGAR, 2 G TOTAL FAT, 3% CALORIES FROM FAT, 0 G SATU-RATED FAT, 7 G FIBER, 297 MG SODIUM

MEXICAN:

1 whole-wheat pita bread

3–4 tablespoons warmed refried beans

1–2 tablespoons low-sodium salsa

1–3 tablespoons corn, thawed if frozen

Vegan Mexican cheese shreds (optional)

1–3 tablespoons guacamole (optional)

Cilantro (optional)

Hot sauce

For a crispy crust, toast the pita or warm in an oven. Warm the refried beans and spread into a thin, even layer on the pita. Add the salsa and corn on top. Sprinkle with cheese shreds, if using. If desired, warm or bake the pizza in a toaster oven for 3 to 5 minutes, until the toppings are warm or the "cheese" has melted. Garnish with guacamole and cilantro before serving, if using. Drizzle with hot sauce, if desired.

PER SERVING (ENTIRE RECIPE): 356 CALORIES, 14 G PROTEIN, 74 G CARBO-HYDRATE, 7 G SUGAR, 4 G TOTAL FAT, 5% CALORIES FROM FAT, 1 G SATU-RATED FAT, 12 G FIBER, 321 MG SODIUM

MEDITERRANEAN:

- 1 whole-wheat pita bread
- 3–4 tablespoons Classic Oil-Free Hummus (page 293) or store-bought hummus
- Balsamic-Dijon Vinaigrette (page 303) or balsamic vinegar
- 1–2 tablespoons diced tomatoes
- 2 tablespoons sliced kalamata olives or black olives
- 2–4 tablespoons chopped spinach or arugula
- 1–2 teaspoons chopped red onion
- 1–2 tablespoons canned chickpeas, rinsed and drained (optional)
- Vegan feta cheese or other vegan cheese (optional)

For a crispy crust, toast pita or warm in an oven, if desired. Prepare the oil-free hummus and balsamic vinaigrette, if using, and set both aside. Spread a thin, even layer of hummus on the pita. Add the tomatoes, olives, and spinach on top, plus onion, chickpeas, and vegan cheese, if using. If desired, warm or bake the pizza in a toaster oven for 3 to 5 minutes, until the toppings are warm or the "cheese" has melted. Drizzle with balsamic vinaigrette before serving.

PER SERVING (ENTIRE RECIPE): 253 CALORIES, 10 G PROTEIN, 42 G CARBO-HYDRATE, 1 G SUGAR, 7 G TOTAL FAT, 8% CALORIES FROM FAT, 1 G SATU-RATED FAT, 8 G FIBER, 574 MG SODIUM

—LN

Neatloaf

SERVES 4	*Easy*

Golden Gravy (page 300) or ketchup, for serving (optional)

1 cup dry lentils

2 cups vegetable broth

1 small onion

1 carrot

1 celery stalk

¼ cup ketchup

2 tablespoons prepared yellow mustard

2 tablespoons low-sodium soy sauce

2 tablespoons nutritional yeast

1 tablespoon Italian seasoning

1 cup instant oats

If using Golden Gravy, prepare and set aside.

Preheat the oven to 350°F. Place a piece of parchment paper in a metal bread pan. Trim the paper so only 2 inches of paper sticks up. Set the pan aside. In a saucepan, combine the lentils with the broth. Cover and bring to a boil. Reduce the heat to low and simmer until the lentils are soft but not mushy and the liquid has evaporated, about 20 minutes.

In a food processor, finely chop the onion, carrot, and celery but do not pulverize them. Transfer to a mixing bowl. Stir in the ketchup, mustard, soy sauce, nutritional yeast, and Italian seasoning; set aside.

Transfer the cooked lentils to a food processor and pulse until most of the lentils are chewed up but some half lentils remain; do not pulverize. Stir the lentils into the prepared mixture. Stir in the oats.

Transfer to the prepared bread pan. Use the back of a spatula or spoon to spread the mixture out evenly and pat down. Bake

40 to 50 minutes, until there is a crisp outer coating. Cover the pan with foil if necessary to prevent burning. Cool in the pan 10 to 15 minutes.

After cooling, place a plate on top of the pan and invert it so the loaf transfers onto the plate. Serve with golden gravy, or ketchup, if using.

PER SERVING (¼ OF RECIPE): 317 CALORIES, 21 G PROTEIN, 49 G CARBO-HYDRATE, 7 G SUGAR, 5 G TOTAL FAT, 7% CALORIES FROM FAT, 19 G FIBER, 58 MG SODIUM

—LN

Vegetable Rice Casserole

SERVES 2 TO 4   *Easy*

1 medium zucchini, diced

5 ounces cherry tomatoes, halved

1 small onion, diced

1 bell pepper (any color), seeded and diced

½ cup vegetable broth, divided

2–5 cloves garlic, minced

1 tablespoon all-purpose flour

1 cup cold soy milk

1½ teaspoons Dijon mustard

1–3 tablespoons nutritional yeast, plus more for garnish (optional)

Salt and pepper

Mrs. Dash Table Seasoning (optional)

2 cups cooked brown rice

½–1 cup canned chickpeas, drained and rinsed, or frozen corn

1 tablespoon chopped fresh basil

2–4 tablespoons breadcrumbs

Vegan Parmesan, optional

Preheat the oven to 425°F. Line a baking sheet with parchment paper. Place the zucchini on the baking sheet in a single layer. Sprinkle the cherry tomatoes, half of the onions, and the bell pepper over the zucchini. Bake 20 to 25 minutes, until the zucchini is roasted and the tomatoes are shriveled.

Meanwhile, pour ¼ cup of the broth into a large skillet. Add the remaining onions and the garlic and sauté until the onions are translucent.

Turn off the heat and add the flour, stirring to evenly coat vegetables. Stir in the cold soy milk and the remaining ¼ cup of broth. Continue stirring until there are no lumps. Cover and bring to a boil. Reduce the heat to low and simmer.

Once the mixture starts to thicken, turn off the heat and stir in the Dijon and nutritional yeast, plus salt and pepper and Mrs. Dash seasoning to taste, if using. Set the sauce aside.

In a glass casserole dish, mix together the cooked rice, oven-roasted vegetables, and chickpeas. Pour the prepared sauce over the top and mix again. Sprinkle with fresh basil and breadcrumbs. Bake for 25 minutes, or until the sauce bubbles and the top is toasty. Garnish with an additional sprinkling of nutritional yeast or vegan Parmesan, if desired.

Note: You can pulverize a slice of stale or toasted bread in a food processor to make breadcrumbs. A combination of corn and chickpeas is also delicious.

PER SERVING (½ OF RECIPE): 290 CALORIES, 16 G PROTEIN, 50 G CARBO-HYDRATE, 14 G SUGAR, 5 G TOTAL FAT, 6% CALORIES FROM FAT, 1 G SATU-RATED FAT, 9 G FIBER, 374 MG SODIUM

—*LN*

Moroccan Shepherd's Pie

SERVES 2   *Elegant*

¼–⅓ cup raisins

2 medium sweet potatoes

1–6 tablespoons soy milk

2 teaspoons ground cumin, divided

1 teaspoon granulated garlic powder

Salt and pepper

½ cup vegetable broth, divided

½ small red onion, diced

1 carrot, diced

2 cloves garlic, minced

1–3 teaspoons minced fresh ginger root

½–1 teaspoon ground cinnamon

½–1 teaspoon chili powder

1 (15-ounce) can lentils, drained and rinsed

¾ cup canned chickpeas or black-eyed peas, drained and rinsed

Preheat the oven to 350°F and set aside a square glass casserole dish. Soak the raisins in boiling hot water for 10 minutes or until plump. Drain and discard the water. Set the raisins aside.

Boil, steam, or pressure-cook the sweet potatoes until very tender. Remove the skin, if desired. Mash the sweet potatoes well, adding soy milk as needed to achieve a "mashed potato" or thick hummus consistency. Stir the ground cumin and garlic powder (to taste; about 1 teaspoon each) into the mashed sweet potatoes, plus a generous amount of salt and pepper, or to taste. Set the mashed sweet potatoes aside.

Pour ¼ cup of the vegetable broth (or water) into a large skillet. Sauté the plumped raisins, onions, carrots, garlic, and ginger until the onions are translucent. Stir in the remaining 1 teaspoon ground cumin, ground cinnamon, and chili powder to coat the vegetables well. Cook for 1 minute. Stir in the lentils, chickpeas, and the remaining ¼ cup of broth. Transfer this mixture to the casserole dish and spread it around evenly. Spread the mashed sweet potatoes evenly over the top. Bake 15 to 40 minutes, until the top is beginning to brown.

Note: Chopped dried apricots or currants may be substituted for raisins; 1 to 2 tablespoons tomato paste can be stirred in with the vegetable filling. For a little crunch, add chopped walnuts to the filling.

PER SERVING (½ OF RECIPE): 326 CALORIES, 11 G PROTEIN, 67 G CARBOHYDRATE, 25 G SUGAR, 3 G TOTAL FAT, 4% CALORIES FROM FAT, 0 G SATURATED FAT, 13 G FIBER, 179 MG SODIUM

—*LN*

Peanut Tofu Stir-Fry

SERVES 2 TO 4 *Easy*

1 (14-ounce) package extra-firm tofu, drained

1 head broccoli, cut into florets

½ cup soy milk

3–4 tablespoons peanut butter

2 tablespoons low-sodium soy sauce

1 tablespoon rice vinegar

1–4 teaspoons chili garlic sauce (e.g., Sambal Oelek; optional)

1 teaspoon maple syrup (optional)

¼ teaspoon granulated garlic powder (optional)

¼ teaspoon ground ginger (optional)

1 teaspoon cornstarch (optional)

1 tablespoon warm water (optional)

Salt and pepper, to taste

Sriracha, for garnish (optional)

Sliced green onions, for garnish (optional)

Sesame seeds, for garnish (optional)

1–2 cups cooked brown rice, for serving (optional)

Wrap the tofu in a clean dish towel and place it between two cutting boards. Place something heavy on the top cutting board to press the tofu for 20 minutes. Unwrap and cube the tofu. If desired, air-fry the tofu cubes at 370°F for 6 minutes, shaking after 3 minutes. For extra crispness, shake again and cook 3 more minutes. Otherwise, skip this step and set the tofu aside.

Steam the broccoli to the desired tenderness; set aside.

In a measuring cup, stir together the soy milk, peanut butter, soy sauce, vinegar, chili garlic sauce, and maple syrup, if using. Add additional chili garlic sauce or maple syrup to taste, if desired. You can also add granulated garlic powder, or ground ginger, if desired.

Transfer the peanut sauce to a small saucepan and heat on low until warm. To thicken it more, whisk 1 teaspoon cornstarch into 1 tablespoon warm water, then stir this cornstarch slurry into the peanut sauce. Heat on low until the sauce thickens; repeat this step if desired. Pour the prepared sauce over the tofu and broccoli or toss it all together. If needed, heat everything in a large skillet or wok on low until thoroughly warm. Season with salt and pepper, if desired. Garnish with sriracha, if desired, and green onions or sesame seeds. Serve with rice, if using.

Note: Red bell peppers or carrots make a nice addition. You can also substitute a bag of frozen stir-fry vegetables; prepare them as directed on the package.

PER SERVING (½ OF RECIPE, EXCLUDING RICE): 101 CALORIES, 8 G PROTEIN, 4 G CARBOHYDRATE, 2 G SUGAR, 7 G TOTAL FAT, 9% CALORIES FROM FAT, 2 G SATURATED FAT, 1 G FIBER, 267 MG SODIUM

—LN

Pasta with Creamy Tofu Sauce

SERVES 4   *Elegant*

Creamy Tofu Sauce (page 304)

10–16 ounces pasta (any variety)

1–2 cups frozen peas (optional)

Black pepper (optional)

Smoked paprika (optional)

Prepare the creamy tofu sauce and set aside. Cook the pasta as directed on the package. If using frozen peas, add them 1 to 2 minutes before the pasta is done cooking. Drain the cooked pasta and peas; do not rinse. Toss the pasta and peas with warmed creamy tofu sauce. Add a sprinkle of black pepper or smoked paprika on top, if desired.

Note: For a spicier dish, garnish with a sprinkle of red pepper flakes. Vegan Parmesan cheese on top is a nice addition. Sun-dried tomatoes can replace peas.

PER SERVING (¼ OF RECIPE): 314 CALORIES, 19 G PROTEIN, 49 G CARBOHYDRATE, 3 G SUGAR, 5 G TOTAL FAT, 3% CALORIES FROM FAT, 1 G SATURATED FAT, 4 G FIBER, 84 MG SODIUM

—*LN*

Nori Rolls with Tahini Dipping Sauce

SERVES 2   *Easy*

Tahini Dipping Sauce (page 305) or hoisin sauce

6 ounces edamame or ⅓ cup hummus

1–4 teaspoons sriracha

1 tablespoon fresh lime juice

1 teaspoon soy sauce (optional)

2 teaspoons warm water

4 sheets nori

½ cup shredded carrot

⅓ Persian cucumber, cut into matchsticks

1 cup chopped spinach

Prepare the tahini dipping sauce, if using, and set aside. If using hoisin sauce, mix with equal parts water and set aside. If using edamame, thaw it and place it in a food processor. Add sriracha, lime juice, soy sauce (if using), and water. Blend into a thick hummus or leave slightly chunky for texture. If using hummus, stir sriracha and lime juice into hummus to taste.

Lay the nori sheets shiny side down. Spread the edamame mixture (or prepared hummus) on the side closest to you. Add vegetables on top, being careful not to overstuff them or the wrap will break. Roll the sheet up. Wet a clean pointer finger and run it along the seam of the nori roll to seal it. Repeat the process. Slice the rolls on the diagonal, if desired. Serve immediately with tahini dipping sauce or prepared hoisin sauce.

Note: Sprouts, cucumber, cilantro, and sliced avocado make a nice addition.

PER SERVING (½ OF RECIPE): 272 CALORIES, 13 G PROTEIN, 19 G CARBO-HYDRATE, 4 G SUGAR, 19 G TOTAL FAT, 24% CALORIES FROM FAT, 3 G SATU-RATED FAT, 6 G FIBER, 332 MG SODIUM

—LN

Potato-Lentil Enchiladas

SERVES 4   *Elegant*

1¾ cups Enchilada Sauce (page 299) or store-bought enchilada
   sauce

1 large sweet potato or russet potato

1–3 teaspoons taco seasoning

1 (15-ounce) can lentils, drained and rinsed

1 cup traditional salsa

4–12 corn tortillas or whole-grain tortillas

Toppings (e.g., vegan cheese, guacamole, sliced olives;
   optional)

Preheat the oven to 350°F. Spritz a 12 x 9-inch casserole baking dish with plant-based oil spray to prevent sticking, if desired. Spread a thin layer of enchilada sauce, about ½ to ¾ cup, on the bottom of the casserole dish and set aside.

Microwave, boil, or steam the sweet potato until fork-tender. Dice or mash the cooked potato. Toss or stir together the prepared potatoes with the taco seasoning to taste. Stir the seasoned potato together with the lentils and salsa; set the mixture aside briefly.

Soften the tortillas in a microwave (see note). Spoon the potato-lentil filling onto a tortilla. Roll it up and place it seam side down in the baking dish. Repeat this process until the filling is used up. Pour the remaining enchilada sauce (about 1 cup) over the rolled tortillas. Cover with foil. Bake until thoroughly warm and the sauce is bubbling, 15 to 20 minutes. If using vegan cheese shreds, add after 10 to 15 minutes.

Garnish with toppings before serving, if desired.

Note: To soften tortillas in a microwave, use a tortilla warming pocket or wrap the tortillas in a damp paper towel; heat 15 to 30 seconds, until pliable.

PER SERVING (¼ OF RECIPE): 279 CALORIES, 13 G PROTEIN, 56 G CARBO-
HYDRATE, 3 G SUGAR, 2 G TOTAL FAT, 3% CALORIES FROM FAT, 14 G FIBER,
535 MG SODIUM

—*LN*

Shroomy Stroganoff

SERVES 4   *Easy*

2 cups Faux Beef Broth (page 306)

8–12 ounces noodles

1–2 cups frozen peas (optional)

16 ounces brown mushrooms, stemmed and sliced

1–2 teaspoons Italian seasoning

1 cup soy milk

¼ cup flour

Black pepper

Garlic powder and onion powder (optional)

Prepare the faux beef broth and set aside. Cook the noodles as directed on the package. If using frozen peas, add them 1 to 2 minutes before the noodles are done. Drain the noodles and peas and set aside.

Pour ¼ cup of the faux beef broth into a large skillet. Add the mushrooms and about 10 shakes of Italian seasoning. Sauté until the mushrooms are soft and have released their juices.

In a measuring cup, whisk together the soy milk, flour, and the remaining faux beef broth. Pour over the cooked mushrooms. Heat on low until the mushroom sauce thickens and is creamy.

Add black pepper to taste, plus garlic and onion powder, to taste, if desired. Toss the mushroom sauce with the cooked noodles and peas, if using. Serve immediately.

Note: For a thicker creamy sauce, stir 1 tablespoon cornstarch into 2 tablespoons water or broth. Whisk together well and add to sauce. Heat on low-medium until it thickens.

PER SERVING (¼ OF RECIPE): 275 CALORIES, 15 G PROTEIN, 46 G CARBOHY-DRATE, 5 G SUGAR, 3 G TOTAL FAT, 4% CALORIES FROM FAT, 1 G SATURATED FAT, 1 G FIBER, 435 MG SODIUM

—LN

Quick Stir-Fry

SERVES 4	*Easy*

2 tablespoons low-sodium soy sauce
1–2 tablespoons coconut sugar or other sugar
1 (16-ounce) bag frozen stir-fry vegetables
½–1 cup cooked rice, for serving
1–2 cups cubed tofu or edamame (optional)
Nuts (e.g., cashews) or sesame seeds (optional)

Whisk together the soy sauce and sugar; set aside. Place the frozen vegetables in a nonstick skillet. Stir and cook until they are warm but still crisp. Re-stir the soy sauce mixture and pour it over the top. Heat for another minute, or until everything is warm. Serve over cooked rice with tofu or edamame, if desired. Garnish with nuts or seeds, if using.

Note: For a more teriyaki-style dish, use 2 tablespoons soy sauce with 1 tablespoon of sugar; the end result is more like a traditional stir-fry dish. For a spicier dish, add sriracha.

PER SERVING (¼ OF RECIPE, EXCLUDING RICE AND TOFU): 147 CALORIES, 10 G PROTEIN, 23 G CARBOHYDRATE, 4 G SUGAR, 3 G TOTAL FAT, 1 G SATU-RATED FAT, 4% CALORIES FROM FAT, 4 G FIBER, 423 MG SODIUM

—LN

Spaghetti and Beanballs

SERVES 2 TO 4 *Easy*

¼ cup vegetable broth or water

½ small onion or 1 shallot, diced

2–3 cloves garlic, minced

2 tablespoons tomato paste

1½ cups cooked brown rice

1 (15-ounce) can navy beans, drained and rinsed

1 teaspoon ketchup

1–2 tablespoons Italian seasoning

1–3 teaspoons dried basil

½ teaspoon red pepper flakes (optional)

1–3 tablespoons breadcrumbs

Salt and pepper

8–16 ounces spaghetti

1 (24-ounce) jar vegan marinara sauce

Pour ¼ cup broth or water into a skillet. Sauté the onions and garlic until the onions are translucent. Add the tomato paste, stirring for 1 minute.

Remove from heat and transfer to a food processor. Add the cooked rice, beans, ketchup, and seasonings to the food processor. Process for 3 to 5 seconds, then stop and scrape the sides. Repeat this process for a total of 10 to 15 seconds. The mixture should be chunky. Stir in the breadcrumbs, plus salt and pepper, about ¼ teaspoon each, or to taste. Add additional seasonings, if desired.

Refrigerate the mixture for at least 30 minutes. Preheat the oven to 350°F. Line a baking sheet with parchment paper. Using clean hands, form the mixture into bouncy ball–size beanballs. Bake for 20 minutes, or until the beanballs are firm to the touch.

Meanwhile, cook the spaghetti as directed on the package and warm the marinara sauce. Toss as much sauce as you like with the cooked spaghetti, then add beanballs on top when serving.

Note: Black beans and kidney beans may be substituted for the navy beans. For a variation or more flavor, add 1 teaspoon ground cumin and ½ teaspoon cayenne pepper. For a more "sausage" flavoring, add ½ teaspoon fennel seeds, or to taste. For a gluten-free option, use 1 to 2 tablespoons chickpea flour instead of breadcrumbs. Vegan Parmesan cheese is also a nice addition to the beanballs!

PER SERVING (½ OF MEATBALL RECIPE, EXCLUDING SPAGHETTI AND SAUCE): 249 CALORIES, 10 G PROTEIN, 46 G CARBOHYDRATE, 5 G SUGAR, 4 G TOTAL FAT, 5% CALORIES FROM FAT, 1 G SATURATED FAT, 9 G FIBER, 99 MG SODIUM

—LN

Aloo Matar (Indian Tomato Potato Curry)

SERVES 2 TO 4 *Easy*

¼ cup vegetable broth

½ small onion, diced

4 cloves garlic, minced

2–3 teaspoons minced fresh ginger root

½ cup tomato sauce

1–2 teaspoons diced green chili (optional)

¼ teaspoon mild curry powder

¼ cup water or vegetable broth

2 medium potatoes, diced

Dash of garam masala

½–1 cup frozen peas

1–4 tablespoons soy milk (optional)

Ketchup (optional)

Salt and pepper

Cooked brown rice or pita bread, for serving

Pour ¼ cup broth into a large pot or deep skillet. Sauté the onions, garlic, green chili, if using, and ginger until the onions are translucent. Transfer to a blender and blend with the tomato sauce. Add the curry powder and ¼ cup water or broth to the blender. Blend briefly to mix everything together.

Transfer back to the saucepan and add the potatoes. Cover and bring to a boil. Reduce the heat to low and simmer until the potatoes are fork-tender, about 10 minutes, stirring periodically. Add a dash or two of garam masala and stir well. Fold in the peas.

Cover and continue to cook on low heat until the peas are warm, adding a splash of water or broth to prevent sticking, if needed. Stir in the soy milk, if using, for a creamier masala. If it is acidic, add a squirt of ketchup (about 1 to 2 tablespoons). Add salt and pepper to taste, plus additional garam masala, if desired. Serve over cooked rice or with whole-wheat pita bread.

Note: You can substitute ¼ to ½ teaspoon ground cumin plus ¾ teaspoon ground coriander for mild curry powder. Garnish with cashews or vegan yogurt and cilantro.

PER SERVING (½ OF RECIPE): 216 CALORIES, 7 G PROTEIN, 48 G CARBOHYDRATE, 8 G SUGAR, 1 G TOTAL FAT, 1% CALORIES FROM FAT, 0 G SATURATED FAT, 9 G FIBER, 365 MG SODIUM

—*LN*

Oven-Baked Macaroni

SERVES 4	*Easy*

1 (12.3-ounce) package silken tofu (e.g., Mori-Nu brand)

2 tablespoons vegetable broth

8 ounces pasta shells

1¼ cups soy milk

½ cup nutritional yeast

1 teaspoon prepared yellow mustard

1 tablespoon granulated onion powder

1 teaspoon granulated garlic powder

½ teaspoon smoked paprika or regular paprika

¼ teaspoon turmeric (for color)

2 tablespoons yellow miso paste

Salt and pepper

¼–½ cup breadcrumbs

Vegan Parmesan or vegan cheddar shreds (optional)

Preheat the oven to 350°F and set aside a glass casserole dish. In a blender, combine the tofu and 2 tablespoons of vegetable broth. Puree until the tofu mixture is smooth and creamy. Set the tofu mixture aside.

Cook the pasta as directed on the package, then drain it and rinse with cold water. Set the cooked pasta aside.

In a saucepan, whisk together the soy milk, nutritional yeast, mustard, and dry spices. Cover and bring almost to a boil. Turn off the heat. Stir in the miso until well combined. Stir in the cooked pasta and tofu mixture until well combined. Season with salt and pepper to taste.

Transfer the mixture to the casserole dish. Sprinkle with breadcrumbs along with vegan Parmesan, if using. Bake 20 to 25 minutes, until the top is slightly browned.

Note: Peas are a nice addition.

PER SERVING (¼ OF RECIPE): 438 CALORIES, 28 G PROTEIN, 69 G CARBOHY-
DRATE, 8 G SUGAR, 7 G TOTAL FAT, 9% CALORIES FROM FAT, 1 G SATURATED
FAT, 9 G FIBER, 518 MG SODIUM

—*LN*

Garlic Cauliflower Risotto

SERVES 2   *Elegant*

½ cup vegetable broth, divided

2–6 cloves garlic, minced

1 (16-ounce) bag frozen riced cauliflower

1 tablespoon water

1 cup soy milk

1–1½ tablespoons flour

1–3 tablespoons nutritional yeast or vegan Parmesan

½ teaspoon granulated onion powder

2 cups cooked brown rice

2–3 cups baby spinach

Salt and pepper (optional)

½ lemon (optional)

Pour ¼ cup of the broth into a skillet. Add the garlic and sauté until most of the liquid has cooked off. Add the riced cauliflower, plus 1 tablespoon water. Cook 5 minutes, stirring regularly, then turn off the heat.

In a small bowl, whisk together the remaining ¼ cup broth, soy milk, flour, nutritional yeast, and granulated onion powder. Pour over the riced cauliflower mixture. Add the cooked brown rice and stir everything together. Turn the heat to high and bring to a near boil. Reduce the heat to low and simmer uncovered until the risotto is creamy and the rice is very soft. Add additional soy milk if needed during simmering.

Turn off the heat and stir in the spinach until it softens into the risotto. Add additional nutritional yeast or vegan Parmesan to taste, plus salt and pepper, if desired. Slice the lemon into 2 wedges and squeeze fresh lemon juice over the top right before serving, if using.

Note: For a richer dish, stir in 1 to 3 teaspoons of tahini or vegan cream cheese to taste.

PER SERVING (½ OF RECIPE): 441 CALORIES, 19 G PROTEIN, 80 G CARBO-HYDRATE, 11 G SUGAR, 7 G TOTAL FAT, 8% CALORIES FROM FAT, 1 G SATU-RATED FAT, 10 G FIBER, 399 MG SODIUM

—LN

Strawberry Banana Nice Cream

SERVES 3   *Convenient*

1½ cups frozen banana
1½ cups frozen strawberries
½ cup unsweetened almond milk
1 teaspoon vanilla extract
Pinch of sea salt

Let the frozen banana and strawberries sit out at room temperature for 10 minutes to thaw slightly.

Add the banana and strawberries, milk, vanilla, and salt to a food processor or high-speed blender and blend until creamy and smooth. If using a blender, start on low and increase the intensity as the fruit starts to puree. Stop as needed to scrape the sides down so everything gets blended.

This is best if served immediately. If it is to be saved for later, transfer it to a container and press plastic wrap to the top of the nice cream before putting a lid on the container. This helps prevent the nice cream from getting icy. Remove it from the freezer and let it sit at room temperature for 5 minutes before enjoying.

PER SERVING (1 CUP): 105 CALORIES, 1 G PROTEIN, 25 G CARBOHYDRATE, 4 G SUGAR, 1 G TOTAL FAT, 1% CALORIES FROM FAT, 0 G SATURATED FAT, 4 G FIBER, 226 MG SODIUM

—*DH*

Beat the Summer Blueberry Pops

SERVES 8 TO 10 *Convenient*

2 cups frozen blueberries

2 bananas, peeled

2 pears, peeled, cores removed, and roughly chopped

½ cup almond milk

Juice of 1 lemon

Add the blueberries, bananas, pears, almond milk, and lemon juice to a blender. Blend until smooth and creamy, then transfer to ice pop molds. Freeze overnight.

Run the molds under warm water to release the ice pops.

PER SERVING (1 POPSICLE): 60 CALORIES, 1 G PROTEIN, 15 G CARBOHYDRATE, 9 G SUGAR, 0 G TOTAL FAT, 0% CALORIES FROM FAT, 0 G SATURATED FAT, 3 G FIBER, 10 MG SODIUM

—*DH*

Triple-Berry No-Churn Sorbet

SERVES 6   *Convenient*

3 cups frozen triple-berry blend

2 bananas

½ cup no-sugar-added cherry juice, pomegranate juice,
    blueberry juice, or cranberry juice, not from concentrate

1–2 tablespoons maple syrup (optional)

Let the berries sit out at room temperature for 5 minutes.

Add the berries, bananas, and juice to a high-speed blender or food processor. If using a blender, start blending on low. Slowly increase the speed until all the fruit is pureed. Continue to blend 1 to 2 minutes, until it is smooth and creamy, stopping to scrape down the sides of the container as needed. Add maple syrup as a sweetener, if desired.

Transfer to a container and press plastic wrap over the top of the sorbet; it should touch the sorbet directly to protect from air and prevent the sorbet from becoming icy. Place a lid on the container and freeze overnight.

Let it sit out at room temperature for 5 to 10 minutes before scooping.

PER SERVING (¾ CUP): 80 CALORIES, 1 G PROTEIN, 21 G CARBOHYDRATE, 12 G SUGAR, 0 G TOTAL FAT, 0% CALORIES FROM FAT, 0 G SATURATED FAT, 4 G FIBER, 2 MG SODIUM

—DH

Lemon Tahini Oat Bites

SERVES 12	*Easy*

2 cups rolled oats, divided
1 cup packed pitted dates
¼ cup tahini
2 tablespoons maple syrup
Juice of 2 lemons
½ teaspoon vanilla extract
⅛ teaspoon sea salt

Add ½ cup of the oats to the food processor bowl and pulse until they are broken down into a coarse flour. Transfer to a small bowl and set aside.

Add the remaining 1½ cups of oats to the food processor and process a few times just to break the oats down into smaller pieces. Do not process into flour—there should still be some texture.

Add the dates, tahini, maple syrup, lemon juice, vanilla, and sea salt and pulse until a sticky dough forms. Form balls using 1 tablespoon of the mixture per ball. Roll the finished balls in the coarse oat flour.

Store in the refrigerator for up to 1 week.

PER SERVING (2 BITES): 133 CALORIES, 3 G PROTEIN, 23 G CARBOHYDRATE, 11 G SUGAR, 4 G TOTAL FAT, 3% CALORIES FROM FAT, 1 G SATURATED FAT, 3 G FIBER, 33 MG SODIUM

—DH

Blueberry Pear Crumble

SERVES 9   *Elegant*

FOR THE FILLING:

3 cups blueberries, fresh or frozen

3 pears, peeled, core removed, and small-diced (at least
    3 cups)

3 tablespoons cornstarch

2 tablespoons maple syrup

Juice of 1 lemon

1 teaspoon vanilla extract

¼ teaspoon sea salt

½ teaspoon ground cinnamon

FOR THE TOPPING:

1½ cups rolled oats

1 teaspoon baking powder

½ teaspoon sea salt

½ teaspoon ground cinnamon

¼ teaspoon ground nutmeg

3 tablespoons maple syrup

3 tablespoons unsweetened almond milk

1 teaspoon vanilla extract

Preheat the oven to 375°F. Line an 8 x 8-inch baking dish with parchment paper.

To make the filling, place the blueberries, pears, and cornstarch in a large bowl and toss to coat the fruit with the cornstarch. Add the maple syrup, lemon juice, vanilla, salt, and cinnamon and stir to combine. Transfer to the prepared baking dish.

To make the topping, add the oats, baking powder, sea salt, cinnamon, and nutmeg to a food processor. Pulse until the mixture is coarse and crumbly. Add the maple syrup, milk, and vanilla. Pulse again a couple of times, just to combine the ingredients. Keep some texture; do not pulverize into flour.

Top the berry-pear mixture evenly with the topping.

Bake for 38 to 42 minutes, until golden brown and bubbling in the center. Remove from the oven, let cool for 10 minutes, cut into 9 pieces, and serve.

PER SERVING (1 PIECE): 146 CALORIES, 2 G PROTEIN, 33 G CARBOHYDRATE, 16 G SUGAR, 1 G TOTAL FAT, 1% CALORIES FROM FAT, 0 G SATURATED FAT, 4 G FIBER, 255 MG SODIUM

—*DH*

Quick Apple Cinnamon Skillet

SERVES 2   *Easy*

3 apples, peeled, core removed, cut into ½-inch chunks
¼ cup water
Juice of ½ lemon
1 tablespoon maple syrup
1 teaspoon ground cinnamon

Heat a nonstick skillet over medium heat. Add the apples and water to the skillet and cook for 6 minutes. Add the lemon juice, maple syrup, and cinnamon. Stir to combine and coat all of the apples while still cooking; cook for 2 more minutes, or until all of the liquid has evaporated. The apples should be fork-tender.

Serve hot or let it cool at room temperature and store in the refrigerator in a tightly sealed container for up to 3 days.

Note: This can also be made with pears; the ripeness of the pears will determine how long you let them cook. Be careful not to let them overcook and turn into mush.

PER SERVING (½ OF RECIPE): 191 CALORIES, 1 G PROTEIN, 51 G CARBO-
HYDRATE, 38 G SUGAR, 1 G TOTAL FAT, 1% CALORIES FROM FAT, 0 G SATU-
RATED FAT, 8 G FIBER, 6 MG SODIUM

—DH

Raspberry Banana Oatmeal Cookies

SERVES 18   *Easy*

2 tablespoons flax meal

¼ cup water

2½ cups rolled oats, divided

1 teaspoon ground cinnamon

½ teaspoon baking soda

½ teaspoon cream of tartar

¼ teaspoon sea salt

2 tablespoons maple syrup

2 teaspoons vanilla extract

½ cup unsweetened applesauce

1 cup mashed banana

1 cup fresh raspberries

Preheat the oven to 350°F. Line a baking sheet with parchment paper.

Combine the flax and water in a small bowl and let it sit for 5 minutes to thicken.

Add 1½ cups of the oats to a blender or food processor and blend into a coarse flour. Be mindful not to process it into a fine flour.

Add the processed oats, remaining oats, cinnamon, baking soda, cream of tartar, and salt to a bowl; whisk to combine. Add the maple syrup, vanilla extract, applesauce, banana, and flax mixture to the bowl and stir to combine. Fold in the raspberries. Do not overmix or the raspberries will start to bleed and the dough will become pink. It is a wet dough.

Use 2 tablespoons of dough to make 1 cookie. Lay the cookies out on the prepared baking sheet 1 inch apart from each other as you make them. Flatten them slightly with the back of a spatula. Wet the back of the spatula with water when flattening the dough if it helps the dough not stick to the spatula.

Bake for 16 to 18 minutes, until the cookies are starting to brown on the bottom. Let them cool on a baking sheet for 10 minutes.

Note: For a Valentine's Day variation, overmix the raspberries so they do start to bleed and the dough turns pink.

PER SERVING (1 COOKIE): 72 CALORIES, 2 G PROTEIN, 14 G CARBOHYDRATE, 4 G SUGAR, 1 G TOTAL FAT, 2% CALORIES FROM FAT, 0 G SATURATED FAT, 2 G FIBER, 70 MG SODIUM

—DH

Black and Blue Brownies

SERVES 16 *Easy*

1 (15.5-ounce) can low-sodium black beans, drained and rinsed
¾ cup all-fruit no-sugar-added blueberry fruit spread, divided
½ cup pitted dates
¼ cup unsweetened applesauce
1 teaspoon vanilla extract
⅛ teaspoon sea salt
½ cup fair-trade unsweetened cocoa powder
¼ cup whole-wheat flour

Preheat the oven to 350°F. Line an 8 x 8-inch baking dish with parchment paper so that the paper overhangs on two sides by a couple of inches.

Add the black beans, ½ cup of the fruit spread, dates, applesauce, vanilla, and sea salt to a food processor and blend until smooth and creamy. Add the cocoa powder and flour and pulse to combine the ingredients. Transfer to the prepared baking dish. Spread the remaining ¼ cup of the fruit spread in a layer on top of the brownie batter.

Bake for 40 to 45 minutes, until the fruit preserves on the top have started to dry slightly. Remove from the oven and let cool completely. Cut into 16 squares.

PER SERVING (1 BROWNIE): 68 CALORIES, 3 G PROTEIN, 15 G CARBOHY-DRATE, 7 G SUGAR, 1 G TOTAL FAT, 2% CALORIES FROM FAT, 0 G SATURATED FAT, 3 G FIBER, 28 MG SODIUM

—DH

Fruity Banana Split

SERVES 1   *Convenient*

1 banana, peeled and sliced in half vertically
½ cup vegan vanilla yogurt
¼ cup sliced strawberries
¼ cup blueberries
Date Caramel Sauce (page 297—optional)
Pomegranate seeds, for garnish (optional)
Fresh mint, for garnish (optional)

Lay the 2 slices of banana on a small plate or in a bowl, side by side. Add the yogurt to the center where the bananas touch, then top with the strawberries and blueberries. Drizzle with date caramel sauce, if using.

Top with a sprinkle of pomegranate seeds and a sprig of fresh mint, if using.

PER SERVING (ENTIRE RECIPE): 241 CALORIES, 4 G PROTEIN, 47 G CARBO-
HYDRATE, 27 G SUGAR, 6 G TOTAL FAT, 3% CALORIES FROM FAT, 0 G SATU-
RATED FAT, 6 G FIBER, 9 MG SODIUM

—DH

Classic Fruit Salad

SERVES 8   *Easy*

2 apples, peeled, cored, and diced

2 bananas, peeled and sliced

Juice of 1 lemon

2 cups hulled and sliced strawberries

2 cups blueberries

1 mango, peeled and cut into chunks

Add the apples, bananas, and lemon juice to a large bowl and toss to combine. Add the strawberries, blueberries, and mango and mix all the ingredients until well combined.

Serve buffet-style or portion into parfait cups.

Note: Create a fruit and yogurt parfait. Use a parfait cup and start with a layer of fruit salad followed by a layer of vegan yogurt, another layer of fruit salad, another layer of yogurt, and finish with a final layer of fruit salad. Garnish with mint, if desired.

PER SERVING (1 CUP): 80 CALORIES, 1 G PROTEIN, 18 G CARBOHYDRATE, 12 G SUGAR, 1 G TOTAL FAT, 2% CALORIES FROM FAT, 0 G SATURATED FAT, 3 G FIBER, 1 MG SODIUM

—DH

Chickpea Cookie Dough Bites

MAKES 18 BITES   *Easy*

1 (15.5-ounce) can low-sodium chickpeas, drained and
      rinsed, or 1½ cups cooked chickpeas
¼ cup almond butter
3 tablespoons maple syrup
1 teaspoon vanilla extract
½ teaspoon sea salt
¼ cup oat flour
5 tablespoons mini vegan chocolate chips

Add the chickpeas, almond butter, maple syrup, vanilla, and sea salt
to a food processor. Process until smooth and creamy. Add the oat
flour and pulse until a dough forms. Add the chocolate chips and
pulse until the chips are evenly dispersed into the dough.

Use a tablespoon or small cookie scoop to scoop out the dough,
1 tablespoon at a time. Roll each scoop into a ball. Refrigerate until
ready to serve.

PER SERVING (2 BITES): 81 CALORIES, 2 G PROTEIN, 10 G CARBOHYDRATE,
4 G SUGAR, 4 G TOTAL FAT, 5% CALORIES FROM FAT, 1 G SATURATED FAT,
2 G FIBER, 138 MG SODIUM

—*DH*

Quickie Cinnamon Rice Pudding

SERVES 4   *Elegant*

---

1 cup cooked brown rice

1½ cups unsweetened almond milk or nondairy milk, divided

2 tablespoons cornstarch

1 teaspoon vanilla extract

1 teaspoon ground cinnamon

Pinch of sea salt

1–2 tablespoons maple syrup (optional)

Add the rice and 1¼ cups of the milk to a saucepot and bring to a boil; reduce the heat to low and let it simmer for 10 minutes, stirring frequently.

Add the remaining ¼ cup milk and cornstarch to a small bowl and whisk to combine and create a slurry. Add the slurry to the pot, stir to combine, and let it simmer for 2 minutes, or until it thickens.

Add the vanilla, cinnamon, and salt and stir to combine. Add maple syrup to make it sweeter, if desired.

Enjoy warm or let it sit in the refrigerator covered for an hour to cool.

PER SERVING (¼ OF RECIPE): 60 CALORIES, 2 G PROTEIN, 15 G CARBOHY-
DRATE, 0 G SUGAR, 1 G TOTAL FAT, 2% CALORIES FROM FAT, 0 G SATURATED
FAT, 1 G FIBER, 117 MG SODIUM

—DH

Carrot Cake

SERVES 8 *Elegant*

¼ cup raisins or walnuts (optional)

1½ cups all-purpose flour or oat flour

½ teaspoon salt

½ teaspoon baking soda

1½ teaspoons ground cinnamon

¼–½ cup brown sugar

1 cup shredded carrots

½ cup crushed pineapple

¼ cup applesauce or vegetable oil

2 teaspoons apple cider vinegar

1–2 teaspoons vanilla extract (optional)

Nondairy milk, as needed

1–2 (8-ounce) packages vegan cream cheese, for frosting

If using raisins, soak them in *hot* water for 10 minutes, or until plump. Drain and reserve the soaking water.

Preheat the oven to 350°F. Spritz an 8-inch square or round pan with plant-based oil spray or use a nonstick pan.

In a large mixing bowl, sift together the flour, salt, baking soda, and ground cinnamon. Stir in the sugar; set aside.

In another bowl, whisk together the carrots, pineapple, applesauce or oil, vinegar, and vanilla, if using. Stir this wet mixture into the dry mixture, then fold in the plumped raisins (or walnuts), if using. If the cake batter is dry (floury) or thick (like hummus), add nondairy milk (or raisin soak water) to moisten. When in doubt, add ¼ cup.

Pour the batter into the prepared pan, patting it down evenly. Bake for 30 minutes, or until a toothpick inserted into the center comes out clean. Allow the cake to cool completely before frosting with vegan cream cheese.

Note: For a sweeter frosting, use electric beaters to whip 1 to 4 table-spoons of confectioners' sugar into room-temperature vegan cream cheese. Orange zest is a nice addition to the cake.

PER SERVING (⅛ OF RECIPE, EXCLUDING CREAM CHEESE): 118 CALORIES, 3 G PROTEIN, 26 G CARBOHYDRATE, 7 G SUGAR, 0 G TOTAL FAT, 0% CALO-RIES FROM FAT, 1 G FIBER, 238 MG SODIUM

—LN

Carrot Cauliflower Cheese Sauce

SERVES 12   *Easy*

1 onion, roughly chopped

2 tablespoons water or vegetable broth

4 cloves garlic, roughly chopped

¼ cup arborio rice

1 medium russet potato, peeled and cut into 1-inch chunks

2 medium carrots, peeled and cut into 1-inch pieces

2 cups cauliflower florets, roughly half a head of cauliflower

3 cups low-sodium vegetable broth

¼ cup nutritional yeast

¼ cup sauerkraut

1 tablespoon white miso paste

1 tablespoon tomato paste

1 tablespoon Dijon mustard

2 teaspoons white wine vinegar

1½ teaspoons sea salt

½ teaspoon smoked paprika

Heat a saucepan over medium heat, add the onion, and sauté for 3 minutes, or until soft. Add the water or vegetable broth as needed to prevent the onion from sticking. Add the garlic and sauté 1 additional minute, or until fragrant, adding liquid if needed. Add the rice, potato, carrots, cauliflower, and vegetable broth. Cover the pot and bring to a boil; reduce to a simmer and let cook for 10 minutes, or until the carrots are fork-tender. Crack the lid, if needed, so it doesn't boil over. Transfer to a blender.

Add the nutritional yeast, sauerkraut, miso, tomato paste, Dijon, vinegar, salt, and smoked paprika to the blender and blend until smooth and creamy.

PER SERVING (½ CUP): 30 CALORIES, 2 G PROTEIN, 6 G CARBOHYDRATE, 6 G SUGAR, 0 G TOTAL FAT, 0% CALORIES FROM FAT, 0 G SATURATED FAT, 1 G FIBER, 117 MG SODIUM

—DH

Creamy Caesar Dressing

SERVES 12   *Easy*

1 (15.5-ounce) can low- sodium great northern beans, drained
    and rinsed, or 1½ cups cooked great northern beans
¼ cup water, plus more as needed
2 tablespoons low-sodium tamari
2 tablespoons Dijon mustard
Juice of 1 lemon
2 cloves garlic
¼ cup nutritional yeast
½ teaspoon sea salt
2 tablespoons capers
½ teaspoon black pepper

Add the beans, water, tamari, Dijon, lemon juice, garlic, nutritional yeast, and salt to a blender and blend until smooth and creamy. Add more water to thin the dressing out, if desired.

Add the capers and pepper and process just until the capers have broken into small bits.

PER SERVING (¼ CUP): 44 CALORIES, 3 G PROTEIN, 6 G CARBOHYDRATE, 0 G SUGAR, 0 G TOTAL FAT, 0% CALORIES FROM FAT, 0 G SATURATED FAT, 2 G FIBER, 306 MG SODIUM

—DH

Power Greens Pesto

SERVES 4 *Easy*

1 cup baby spinach

1 cup torn curly kale, stems removed

1 cup basil leaves, packed

¼ cup nutritional yeast

¼ cup vegetable broth

Juice of ½ lemon

1 teaspoon white miso paste

1 clove garlic

½ teaspoon sea salt

¼ teaspoon ground black pepper

Add the spinach, kale, basil, nutritional yeast, vegetable broth, lemon juice, miso, garlic, salt, and pepper to a food processor and process until smooth and creamy.

PER SERVING (¼ OF RECIPE): 37 CALORIES, 4 G PROTEIN, 5 G CARBOHY-DRATE, 1 G SUGAR, 0 G TOTAL FAT, 0% CALORIES FROM FAT, 0 G SATURATED FAT, 2 G FIBER, 389 MG SODIUM

—DH

Classic Oil-Free Hummus

SERVES 6   *Convenient*

1 (15.5-ounce) can low-sodium chickpeas, drained and
    rinsed, or 1½ cups cooked chickpeas
¼ cup water
2 tablespoons tahini (optional)
1 clove garlic
Juice of 1 lemon
¼ teaspoon ground cumin
¼ teaspoon sea salt
Smoked paprika, for garnish (optional)

Add the chickpeas, water, tahini, if using, garlic, lemon juice, cumin, and salt to a food processor and process until smooth and creamy. Garnish with smoked paprika, if desired.

Note: Add ¾ cup roasted red peppers from a jar for a roasted red pepper hummus; simply puree with all the other ingredients in the food processor. You can also add ¾ cup of the power greens pesto (page 292) for a pesto hummus.

PER SERVING (¼ CUP): 63 CALORIES, 4 G PROTEIN, 12 G CARBOHYDRATE, 0 G SUGAR, 1 G TOTAL FAT, 2% CALORIES FROM FAT, 0 G SATURATED FAT, 4 G FIBER, 168 MG SODIUM

—DH

White Bean Tzatziki

SERVES 6 *Makes 1 ½ cups*

---

1 (15.5-ounce) can low-sodium great northern beans, drained
   and rinsed
½ cup water
Juice of 1 lemon
1 teaspoon garlic powder
½ teaspoon sea salt
½ cup grated cucumber
3 tablespoons finely chopped fresh dill

Add the beans, water, lemon juice, garlic, and salt to a blender. Blend until smooth and creamy. Transfer to a bowl.

Wrap the grated cucumber in a paper towel and squeeze any of the excess water out over a sink. Add the cucumber and dill to the bowl with the bean mixture and stir to combine the ingredients. Transfer to a container with an airtight lid. It will keep in the refrigerator for up to 5 days.

PER SERVING (¼ CUP): 66 CALORIES, 4 G PROTEIN, 11 G CARBOHYDRATE, 1 G SUGAR, 1 G TOTAL FAT, 2% CALORIES FROM FAT, 0 G SATURATED FAT, 3 G FIBER, 238 MG SODIUM

—*DH*

Cinnamon Blueberry Syrup

SERVES 4   *Easy*

1½ cups fresh or frozen blueberries, thawed if frozen

½ teaspoon vanilla extract

½ teaspoon ground cinnamon

Maple syrup (optional)

Add the blueberries, vanilla, and cinnamon to a blender. Start the blender on low and increase the speed as all of the berries are pureed. Blend until smooth and creamy.

Taste for sweetness, and add maple syrup, if desired, to taste. Add water, if desired, for a thinner consistency.

PER SERVING (¼ CUP): 35 CALORIES, 0 G PROTEIN, 8 G CARBOHYDRATE, 5 G SUGAR, 0 G TOTAL FAT, 0% CALORIES FROM FAT, 0 G SATURATED FAT, 2 G FIBER, 1 MG SODIUM

—DH

Chimichurri Sauce

SERVES 4   *Easy*

---

1 cup chopped fresh parsley

4 cloves garlic

1 medium red chili pepper or ½ serrano pepper, seeds
    removed and roughly chopped

1 teaspoon paprika

½ teaspoon dried oregano

½ teaspoon sea salt

¼ teaspoon ground black pepper

¼ cup red wine vinegar

Juice of ½ lemon

Add the parsley, garlic, chili, paprika, oregano, salt, pepper, vinegar, and lemon juice to a food processor. Process until all the ingredients have broken down into a thick paste-like consistency. There will be some liquid separation; stir before use.

Note: Use crushed red pepper flakes, to taste, as a substitute for the chili or pepper, if needed.

PER SERVING (¼ CUP): 20 CALORIES, 1 G PROTEIN, 3 G CARBOHYDRATE, 1 G SUGAR, 0 G TOTAL FAT, 0% CALORIES FROM FAT, 0 G SATURATED FAT, 1 G FIBER, 293 MG SODIUM

—DH

Oil-Free Crispy Chickpea Croutons

SERVES 8 *Easy*

1 cup dry chickpeas, soaked in water overnight, drained and rinsed
Juice of ½ lemon
2 tablespoons nutritional yeast
1 teaspoon sea salt
1 teaspoon garlic powder
1 teaspoon onion powder

Preheat the oven to 375°F. Line a baking sheet with parchment paper.

Add the chickpeas and lemon juice to a bowl and toss to combine. Add the nutritional yeast, salt, garlic powder, and onion powder. Toss everything to coat the chickpeas with the dry spices. Transfer the seasoned chickpeas to the prepared baking sheet.

Bake for 20 minutes, toss, and bake an additional 10 minutes, or until the chickpeas have started to crisp up slightly and all of the chickpeas are dry.

Let them cool. Use the croutons on salad or in bowls as desired.

PER SERVING (2 TABLESPOONS): 102 CALORIES, 6 G PROTEIN, 17 G CARBO-
HYDRATE, 3 G SUGAR, 2 G TOTAL FAT, 2% CALORIES FROM FAT, 0 G SATU-
RATED FAT, 3 G FIBER, 300 MG SODIUM

—DH

Date Caramel Sauce

SERVES 8   *Easy*

1 cup pitted and chopped Medjool dates, soaked in warm
    water for 10 minutes and drained
¾ cup water
1 teaspoon vanilla extract
½ teaspoon ground cinnamon
Pinch of sea salt

Add the dates, water, vanilla, cinnamon, and salt to a blender and
process until smooth and creamy. Add water, 1 tablespoon at a time,
as needed for a thinner consistency.

PER SERVING (2 TABLESPOONS): 58 CALORIES, 1 G PROTEIN, 13 G CARBO-
HYDRATE, 3 G SUGAR, 0 G TOTAL FAT, 0% CALORIES FROM FAT, 0 G SATU-
RATED FAT, 1 G FIBER, 19 MG SODIUM

—DH

Easy Arrabbiata Sauce

SERVES 7

4 cloves garlic, minced

2 teaspoons crushed red pepper

3 tablespoons tomato paste

1 (28-ounce) can crushed tomatoes

1 tablespoon maple syrup

½ teaspoon sea salt

Heat a nonstick saucepot over medium heat. Add the garlic and crushed red pepper and sauté for 1 minute, or until fragrant. Use water, 2 tablespoons at a time, to prevent the garlic from sticking or burning. Add the tomato paste and stir together with the garlic and crushed red pepper until combined; cook for about 3 minutes, until the tomato paste turns darker in color. Use water as needed to prevent the ingredients from sticking or burning.

Add the crushed tomatoes, maple syrup, and salt and stir to combine. Lower the heat and let simmer, uncovered, for 20 minutes, or until the flavors have become richer and spicier. Taste and adjust as needed, adding more crushed red pepper to increase the heat and maple syrup to lessen the intensity of the heat.

Crushed red pepper intensity varies; if you know you have a very spicy variety, start with 1 teaspoon of crushed red pepper and adjust from there.

Serve hot with pasta and vegetables, as desired.

PER SERVING (½ CUP): 47 CALORIES, 2 G PROTEIN, 9 G CARBOHYDRATE, 6 G SUGAR, 0 G TOTAL FAT, 0% CALORIES FROM FAT, 0 G SATURATED FAT, 2 G FIBER, 362 MG SODIUM

—*DH*

Enchilada Sauce

SERVES 2 TO 4 *Easy*

1 cup vegetable broth or water

1 (8-ounce) can tomato sauce

2 tablespoons cornstarch

1–2 tablespoons chili powder

¼ teaspoon granulated garlic powder

⅛ teaspoon granulated onion powder

¼ teaspoon ground cumin (optional)

In a saucepan, whisk together all the ingredients. Taste, adding ground cumin, if using, or other spices.

Note: For a "chipotle" version, stir adobo sauce into the enchilada sauce to taste or use chipotle powder to taste.

PER SERVING (ENTIRE RECIPE): 169 CALORIES, 2 G PROTEIN, 39 G CARBO-HYDRATE, 12 G SUGAR, 2 G TOTAL FAT, 2% CALORIES FROM FAT, 0 G SATU-RATED FAT, 8 G FIBER, 188 MG SODIUM

—LN

Golden Gravy

SERVES 1 TO 2	*Elegant*

1 cup vegetable broth, divided

1 small onion, thinly sliced

⅓ teaspoon granulated onion powder

1½ tablespoons nutritional yeast

1½ tablespoons low-sodium soy sauce

1–2 teaspoons Dijon mustard

1 tablespoon cornstarch

1 tablespoon chickpea flour

Dash of granulated garlic powder

Salt and pepper

Mrs. Dash All-Purpose Seasoning (optional)

Pour ¼ cup of the broth into a skillet. Sauté the onion until translucent and very soft, adding water or more broth, if needed.

In a small bowl, whisk the granulated onion powder, nutritional yeast, soy sauce, Dijon, cornstarch, chickpea flour, and granulated garlic powder into the remaining ¾ cup broth. Pour the mixture over the onions. Heat on low until the gravy is thick and warm, stirring occasionally. Add salt and pepper to taste, plus a few dashes of Mrs. Dash seasoning, if using.

PER SERVING (ENTIRE RECIPE): 148 CALORIES, 1 G PROTEIN, 28 G CARBOHYDRATE, 4 G SUGAR, 1 G TOTAL FAT, 1% CALORIES FROM FAT, 0 G SATURATED FAT, 6 G FIBER, 133 MG SODIUM

—LN

Barbecue Sauce

SERVES 8   *Convenient*

1 (8-ounce) can tomato sauce

1–3 tablespoons maple syrup or brown sugar

1 teaspoon Dijon mustard

Dash of chili powder

½ teaspoon granulated onion powder

¼–½ teaspoon granulated garlic powder

1 tablespoon tomato paste (optional)

1 tablespoon apple cider vinegar (optional)

½ teaspoon smoked paprika (optional)

Dash of cayenne pepper or chipotle powder (optional)

Salt and pepper (optional)

In a saucepan, whisk together the tomato sauce, 1 tablespoon of the maple syrup, Dijon mustard, chili powder, onion powder, and garlic powder. Add more maple syrup to taste. Add optional ingredients as desired to taste. Heat the sauce on low until thoroughly warm. If using for the Cauliflower BBQ Sliders (page 195), you do not need to heat the sauce.

Note: For a Kansas City–style sauce, add 1 to 2 teaspoons vegan Worcestershire sauce and 1 to 2 tablespoons molasses (not black-strap). Heat on low, if desired.

PER SERVING (APPROXIMATELY 2 TABLESPOONS, ⅛ OF RECIPE): 19 CALO-RIES, 1 G PROTEIN, 5 G CARBOHYDRATE, 3 G SUGAR, 0 G TOTAL FAT, 0% CALORIES FROM FAT, 0 G SATURATED FAT, 1 G FIBER, 12 MG SODIUM

—LN

Low-Fat Vegan Mayo

SERVES 30 *Convenient*

1 (12.3-ounce) package silken tofu (e.g., Mori-Nu brand)

1–3 teaspoons Dijon mustard

1–2 tablespoons fresh lemon juice or red wine vinegar

¼ teaspoon agave nectar or maple syrup

¼ teaspoon granulated garlic powder (optional)

Salt

In a small blender or mini food processor, combine all the ingredients, starting with the least amount of mustard and lemon juice. Blend well. Add additional mustard, lemon juice, and agave nectar, plus salt, to taste.

PER SERVING (1 TABLESPOON): 10 CALORIES, 1 G PROTEIN, 1 G CARBOHYDRATE, 0 G SUGAR, 0 G TOTAL FAT, 0 G SATURATED FAT, 0 G FIBER, 8 MG SODIUM

—*LN*

Mango Salsa

SERVES 2 TO 6 *Easy*

1–4 tablespoons finely diced red onion

2 mangoes

1 small Persian cucumber, diced (optional)

1–3 tablespoons finely chopped cilantro or fresh mint, stemmed

2 tablespoons white balsamic vinegar or mango vinegar

Juice of 1 small lime (optional)

Salt and pepper (optional)

½ avocado (optional)

Soak the onion in cold water for 5 minutes; drain. Remove the skin from the mangoes and carefully cut the mango flesh away from the large pit. Dice small and set aside.

If using a cucumber, remove the skin and dice small. In a mixing bowl, toss together the onion, mango, cilantro or mint, and vinegar, plus the cucumber and lime juice, if using. Add salt and pepper to taste, if desired. Chill for 15 minutes, or longer if you can. If using avocado, dice it small and mix it in immediately before serving or it may brown.

Note: For a spicy version, add 1 to 2 teaspoons minced habanero or jalapeño pepper. If you can't find a Persian cucumber (they are much smaller than "regular" cucumbers), remove skin and seeds from a regular cucumber, then dice it. Soaking onions first mellows the onion flavor and helps retain their crunch.

PER SERVING (ENTIRE RECIPE, EXCLUDING AVOCADO): 414 CALORIES, 6 G PROTEIN, 102 G CARBOHYDRATE, 93 G SUGAR, 3 G TOTAL FAT, 3% CALORIES FROM FAT, 1 G SATURATED FAT, 11 G FIBER, 12 MG SODIUM

—LN

Balsamic-Dijon Vinaigrette

SERVES 1 *Easy*

⅓ cup balsamic vinegar
1–3 tablespoons Dijon mustard
1–3 teaspoons nutritional yeast
½ teaspoon Italian seasoning (optional)
Maple syrup, to taste (optional)

Whisk together all the ingredients. Adjust to taste.

PER SERVING (ENTIRE RECIPE): 39 CALORIES, 2 G PROTEIN, 3 G CARBOHY-
DRATE, 1 G SUGAR, 1 G TOTAL FAT, 1% CALORIES FROM FAT, 0 G SATURATED
FAT, 1 G FIBER, 183 MG SODIUM

—LN

Creamy Tofu Sauce

SERVES 4 *Easy*

---

1 (12.3-ounce) package silken tofu (e.g., Mori-Nu brand)
2½–3 tablespoons nutritional yeast or vegan Parmesan
Juice of 1 medium lemon (1–2 tablespoons juice)
1 teaspoon granulated garlic powder
½–1 teaspoon granulated onion powder
1–2 tablespoons soy milk or other nondairy milk (optional)
Salt and pepper (optional)

In a blender, combine the tofu, nutritional yeast, lemon juice, and spices. Blend until smooth and creamy, adding soy milk as needed or desired. Add salt and pepper to taste, if desired. Transfer to a saucepan and heat over low until warm.

PER SERVING (¼ OF RECIPE): 72 CALORIES, 8 G PROTEIN, 5 G CARBOHY-
DRATE, 2 G SUGAR, 3 G TOTAL FAT, 3% CALORIES FROM FAT, 0 G SATURATED
FAT, 1 G FIBER, 33 MG SODIUM

—LN

Orange Ginger Dressing

SERVES 1   *Easy*

1–2 tablespoons warm water

2 tablespoons orange marmalade

1½ teaspoons rice vinegar

1½ teaspoons low-sodium soy sauce

Dash of ground ginger

Sriracha

Whisk together all the ingredients. Adjust to taste.

PER SERVING (ENTIRE RECIPE): 107 CALORIES, 1 G PROTEIN, 27 G CARBO-
HYDRATE, 25 G SUGAR, 0 G TOTAL FAT, 0% CALORIES FROM FAT, 0 G SATU-
RATED FAT, 0 G FIBER, 462 MG SODIUM

—LN

Tahini Dipping Sauce

SERVES 1   *Easy*

¼ cup tahini

1 teaspoon miso paste

1 teaspoon low-sodium soy sauce

Juice of 1 small lime

½ teaspoon maple syrup

1 tablespoon vegetable broth or water

Whisk together all the ingredients. Taste and adjust (e.g., add
another ½ teaspoon miso, soy sauce, and/or lime juice). Thin with
additional broth or water, if desired.

PER SERVING (ENTIRE RECIPE): 384 CALORIES, 11 G PROTEIN, 19 G CAR-
BOHYDRATE, 3 G SUGAR, 33 G TOTAL FAT, 42% CALORIES FROM FAT, 5 G
SATURATED FAT, 6 G FIBER, 577 MG SODIUM

—LN

Faux Beef Broth

SERVES 2   *Easy*

---

2 cups water

2 tablespoons low-sodium soy sauce

2 tablespoons nutritional yeast

½ teaspoon granulated onion powder

½ teaspoon granulated garlic powder

Dash of ground ginger

1 teaspoon vegan Worcestershire sauce (optional)

Whisk together all the ingredients.

PER SERVING (HALF OF RECIPE): 10 CALORIES, 2 G PROTEIN, 2 G CARBOHY-
DRATE, 0 G SUGAR, 0 G TOTAL FAT, 0% CALORIES FROM FAT, 0 G SATURATED
FAT, 1 G FIBER, 224 MG SODIUM

—LN

Creamy Garlic Yogurt Sauce

SERVES 1 TO 2   *Easy*

---

1 teaspoon minced garlic

6 ounces plain, unsweetened vegan yogurt

1–3 teaspoons water (optional)

Salt and pepper (optional)

Stir the garlic into the yogurt until well combined. Add water, 1 teaspoon at a time, to thin the sauce to the desired consistency. Add salt and pepper to taste, if desired.

PER SERVING (ENTIRE RECIPE): 125 CALORIES, 10 G PROTEIN, 13 G CARBO-
HYDRATE, 12 G SUGAR, 2 G TOTAL FAT, 3% CALORIES FROM FAT, 0 G FIBER,
120 MG SODIUM

—LN

Notes

Introduction

1. Barnard ND, Scialli AR, Turner-McGrievy G, Lanou AJ, Glass J. "The effects of a low-fat, plant-based dietary intervention on body weight, metabolism, and insulin sensitivity." *American Journal of Medicine* 2005;118:991–997.
2. Karl JP, Meydani M, Barnett JB, et al. "Substituting whole grains for refined grains in a 6-wk randomized trial favorably affects energy-balance metrics in healthy men and postmenopausal women." *American Journal of Clinical Nutrition* 2017;105:589–599.
3. Kahleova H, Petersen KF, Shulman GI, et al. "Effect of a low-fat vegan diet on body weight, insulin sensitivity, postprandial metabolism, and intramyocellular and hepatocellular lipids in overweight adults: a randomized clinical trial." *JAMA Network Open* 2020. Nov 2;3(11):e2025454.

Chapter 1. The Breakthroughs and What They Mean for You

1. Barnard ND, Scialli AR, Turner-McGrievy G, Lanou AJ, Glass J. "The effects of a low-fat, plant-based dietary intervention on body weight, metabolism, and insulin sensitivity." *American Journal of Medicine* 2005;118:991–997.
2. Mishra S, Xu J, Agarwal U, Gonzales J, Levin S, Barnard N. "A multicenter randomized controlled trial of a plant-based nutrition program to reduce body weight and cardiovascular risk in the corporate setting: the GEICO study." *European Journal of Clinical Nutrition* 2013;67:718–724.
3. Barnard ND, Alwarith J, Rembert E, et al. "A Mediterranean diet and low-fat vegan diet to improve body weight and cardiometabolic risk factors: a randomized, cross-over trial." *Journal of the American Nutrition Association* 2021 Feb 5:1–13.
4. Whiting S, Derbyshire EJ, Tiwari B. "Could capsaicinoids help to support weight management? A systematic review and meta-analysis of energy intake data." *Appetite* 2014;73:183–188.
5. Mueller-Cunningham WM, Quintana R, Kasim-Karakas SE. "An ad libitum, very low-fat diet results in weight loss and changes in nutrient intakes in postmenopausal women." *Journal of the American Dietetic Association* 2003;103:1600–1606.
6. Astrup A, Astrup A, Buemann B, Flint A, Raben A. "Low-fat diets and energy

balance: how does the evidence stand in 2002?" *Proceedings of the Nutrition Society* 2002;61:299–309.

7. Karl JP, Meydani M, Barnett JB, et al. "Substituting whole grains for refined grains in a 6-wk randomized trial favorably affects energy-balance metrics in healthy men and postmenopausal women." *American Journal of Clinical Nutrition* 2017;105:589–599; Schlesinger S, Neuenschwander M, Schwedhelm C, et al. "Food groups and risk of overweight, obesity, and weight gain: a systematic review and dose-response meta-analysis of prospective studies." *Advances in Nutrition* 2019;10:205–218.

8. Sparks LM, Xie H, Koza RA, et al. "A high-fat diet coordinately downregu-lates genes required for mitochondrial oxidative phosphorylation in skeletal muscle." *Diabetes* 2005;54:1926–1933.

9. Anderson AS, Haynie KR, McMillan RP, et al. "Early skeletal muscle adapta-tions to short-term high-fat diet in humans before changes in insulin sensitiv-ity." *Obesity* 2015;23:720–724.

10. Jennings A, MacGregor A, Spector T, Cassidy A. "Higher dietary flavonoid intakes are associated with lower objectively measured body composition in women: evidence from discordant monozygotic twins." *American Journal of Clinical Nutrition* 2017;105:626–634.

11. Bertoia ML, Mukamal KJ, Cahill LE, et al. "Changes in intake of fruits and vegetables and weight change in United States men and women followed for up to 24 years: analysis from three prospective cohort studies." *PLoS Medicine* 12(9):e1001878; Bertoia ML, Rimm EB, Mukamal KJ, Hu FB, Willett WC, Cassidy A. "Dietary flavonoid intake and weight maintenance: three prospec-tive cohorts of 124 086 US men and women followed for up to 24 years." *Brit-ish Medical Journal* 2016;352:i17.

12. Rao PV, Gan SH. "Cinnamon: a multifaceted medicinal plant." *Evidence-Based Complementary and Alternative Medicine* 2014;2014:642942.

13. Jain SG, Puri S, Misra A, Gulati S, Mani K. "Effect of oral cinnamon interven-tion on metabolic profile and body composition of Asian Indians with meta-bolic syndrome: a randomized double-blind control trial." *Lipids in Health and Disease* 2017;16:113.

14. Kahleova H, Petersen KF, Shulman GI, et al. "Effect of a low-fat vegan diet on body weight, insulin sensitivity, postprandial metabolism, and intramyocellu-lar and hepatocellular lipids in overweight adults: a randomized clinical trial." *JAMA Network Open* 2020. Nov 2;3(11):e2025454.

Chapter 2. The Best Foods for Powering Your Weight Loss

1. Rao PV, Gan SH. "Cinnamon: a multifaceted medicinal plant." *Evidence-Based Complementary and Alternative Medicine* 2014;2014:642942; Jain SG, Puri S, Misra A, Gulati S, Mani K. "Effect of oral cinnamon intervention on metabolic profile and body composition of Asian Indians with metabolic syndrome: a randomized double-blind control trial." *Lipids in Health and Disease* 2017;16:113.

2. Keramati M, Musazadeh V, Malekahmadi M, et al. "Cinnamon, an effective anti-obesity agent: evidence from an umbrella meta-analysis." *Journal of Food Biochemistry* 2022 Aug;46(8):e14166.

3. Whiting S, Derbyshire EJ, Tiwari B. "Could capsaicinoids help to support weight management? A systematic review and meta-analysis of energy intake data." *Appetite* 2014;73:183–188.

4. Snitker S, Fujishima Y, Shen H, et al. "Effects of novel capsinoid treatment on fatness and energy metabolism in humans: possible pharmacogenetic implications." *American Journal of Clinical Nutrition* 2009;89(1):45–50.

5. Saito M, Yoneshiro T. "Capsinoids and related food ingredients activating brown fat thermogenesis and reducing body fat in humans." *Current Opinion in Lipidology* 2013;24:71–77; Yoneshiro T, Aita S, Kawai Y, Iwanaga T, Saito M. "Nonpungent capsaicin analogs (capsinoids) increase energy expenditure through the activation of brown adipose tissue in humans." *American Journal of Clinical Nutrition* 2012;95:845–850; Tremblay A, Arguin H, Panahi S. "Capsaicinoids: a spicy solution to the management of obesity? *International Journal of Obesity (London)* 2016;40:1198–1204; Inoue N, Matsunaga Y, Satoh H, Takahashi M. "Enhanced energy expenditure and fat oxidation in humans with high BMI scores by the ingestion of novel and non-pungent capsaicin analogues (capsinoids)." *Bioscience, Biotechnology, and Biochemistry* 2007;71:380–389.

6. Ohnuki K, Niwa S, Maeda S, Inoue N, Yazawa S, Fushiki T. "CH-19 sweet, a non-pungent cultivar of red pepper, increased body temperature and oxygen consumption in humans." *Bioscience, Biotechnology, and Biochemistry* 2001;65:2033–2036; Hachiya S, Kawabata F, Ohnuki K, et al. "Effects of CH-19 Sweet, a non-pungent cultivar of red pepper, on sympathetic nervous activity, body temperature, heart rate, and blood pressure in humans." *Bioscience, Biotechnology, and Biochemistry* 2007;71:671–676.

7. Maharlouei N, Tabrizi R, Lankarani KB, et al. "The effects of ginger intake on weight loss and metabolic profiles among overweight and obese subjects: a systematic review and meta-analysis of randomized controlled trials." *Critical Reviews in Food Science and Nutrition* 2019;59(11):1753–1766.

8. Bertoia ML, Mukamal KJ, Cahill LE, et al. "Changes in intake of fruits and vegetables and weight change in United States men and women followed for up to 24 years: analysis from three prospective cohort studies." *PLoS Medicine* 12(9):e1001878; Bertoia ML, Rimm EB, Mukamal KJ, Hu FB, Willett WC, Cassidy A. "Dietary flavonoid intake and weight maintenance: three prospective cohorts of 124 086 US men and women followed for up to 24 years." *British Medical Journal* 2016;352:i17; Jennings A, MacGregor A, Spector T, Cassidy A. "Higher dietary flavonoid intakes are associated with lower objectively measured body composition in women: evidence from discordant monozygotic twins." *American Journal of Clinical Nutrition* 2017;105:626–634.

9. Krikorian R, Shidler MD, Nash TA, et al. "Blueberry supplementation improves memory in older adults." *Journal of Agricultural and Food Chemistry* 2010;58:3996–4000.

10. Krikorian R, Nash TA, Shidler MD, Shukitt-Hale B, Joseph JA. "Concord grape juice supplementation improves memory function in older adults with mild cognitive impairment." *British Journal of Nutrition* 2010;103:730–734.

11. Travica N, D'Cunha NM, Naumovski N, et al. "The effect of blueberry interventions on cognitive performance and mood: a systematic review of randomized controlled trials." *Brain, Behavior, and Immunity* 2020;85:96–105; Agarwal P, Holland TH, James BD, et al. "Pelargonidin and berry intake association with Alzheimer's disease neuropathology: a community-based study." *Journal of Alzheimer's Disease* 2022;88:653–661.

12. De Oliveira MC, Sichieri R, Venturim Mozzer R. "A low-energy-dense diet adding fruit reduces weight and energy intake in women." *Appetite* 2008;51:291–295.

13. Chai SC, Hooshmand S, Saadat RL, Payton ME, Brummel-Smith K, Arjmandi BH. "Daily apple versus dried plum: impact on cardiovascular disease risk factors in postmenopausal women." *Journal of the Academy of Nutrition and Dietetics* 2012;112:1158–1168.

14. Barth SW, Koch TC, Watzl B, Dietrich H, Will F, Bub A. "Moderate effects of apple juice consumption on obesity-related markers in obese men: impact of diet-gene interaction on body fat content." *European Journal of Nutrition* 2012;51:841–850.

15. Coronel J, Pinos I, Amengual J. "β-carotene in obesity research: technical considerations and current status of the field." *Nutrients* 2019;11(4):842.

16. Brady WE, Mares-Perlman JA, Bowen P, Stacewicz-Sapuntzakis M. "Human serum carotenoid concentrations are related to physiologic and lifestyle factors." *Journal of Nutrition* 1996;126:129–137.

17. Canas JA, Lochrie A, McGowan AG, Hossain J, Schettino C, Balagopal PB. "Effects of mixed carotenoids on adipokines and abdominal adiposity in children: a pilot study." *Journal of Clinical Endocrinology and Metabolism* 2017;102:1983–1990.

18. Morris MC, Evans EA, Bienias JL, et al. "Dietary fats and the risk of incident Alzheimer's disease." *Archives of Neurology* 2003;60:194–200.

19. Neelakantan N, Seah JYH, van Dam RM. "The effect of coconut oil consumption on cardiovascular risk factors: a systematic review and meta-analysis of clinical trials." *Circulation* 2020;141:803–814.

20. Sun Y, Neelakantan N, Wu Y, Lote-Oke R, Pan A, van Dam RM. "Palm oil consumption increases LDL cholesterol compared with vegetable oils low in saturated fat in a meta-analysis of clinical trials." *Journal of Nutrition* 2015;145:1549–1558.

21. Li SS, Kendall CW, de Souza RJ, et al. "Dietary pulses, satiety and food intake: a systematic review and meta-analysis of acute feeding trials." *Obesity* (Silver Spring) 2014;22:1773–1780.

22. Kim SJ, de Souza RJ, Choo VL, et al. "Effects of dietary pulse consumption on body weight: a systematic review and meta-analysis of randomized controlled trials." *American Journal of Clinical Nutrition* 2016;103:1213–1223.

23. Jenkins DJ, Mirrahimi A, Srichaikul K, et al. "Soy protein reduces serum

cholesterol by both intrinsic and food displacement mechanisms." *Journal of Nutrition* 2010;140:2302S–2311S.

24. Xie Q, Chen ML, Qin Y, et al. "Isoflavone consumption and risk of breast cancer: a dose-response meta-analysis of observational studies." *Asia Pacific Journal of Clinical Nutrition* 2013;22:118–127; Chen M, Rao Y, Zheng Y, et al. "Association between soy isoflavone intake and breast cancer risk for pre- and post-menopausal women: a meta-analysis of epidemiological studies." *PLoS ONE* 2014;9(2):e89288.

25. Nechuta SJ, Caan BJ, Chen WY, et al. "Soy food intake after diagnosis of breast cancer and survival: an in-depth analysis of combined evidence from cohort studies of US and Chinese women." *American Journal of Clinical Nutrition* 2012;96:123–132; Chi F, Wu R, Zeng YC, Xing R, Liu Y, Xu ZG. "Post-diagnosis soy food intake and breast cancer survival: a meta-analysis of cohort studies." *Asian Pacific Journal of Cancer Prevention* 2013;14:2407–2412.

26. Barnard ND, Kahleova H, Holtz DN, et al. "A dietary intervention for vaso-motor symptoms of menopause: a randomized, controlled trial." *Menopause* 2023;30(1):80–87.

27. Jenkins DJ, Kendall CW, Marchie A, et al. "Direct comparison of a dietary portfolio of cholesterol-lowering foods with a statin in hypercholesterolemic participants." *American Journal of Clinical Nutrition* 2005;81:380–387.

28. Karl JP, Meydani M, Barnett JB, et al. "Substituting whole grains for refined grains in a 6-wk randomized trial favorably affects energy-balance metrics in healthy men and postmenopausal women." *American Journal of Clinical Nutrition* 2017;105:589–599.

29. Ye EQ, Chacko SA, Chou EL, Kugizaki M, Liu S. "Greater whole-grain intake is associated with lower risk of type 2 diabetes, cardiovascular disease, and weight gain." *Journal of Nutrition* 2012;142:1304–1313.

30. Zhang R, Zhang X, Wu K, et al. "Rice consumption and cancer incidence in US men and women." *International Journal of Cancer* 2016;138:555–564.

31. Chiavaroli L, Kendall CWC, Braunstein CR, et al. "Effect of pasta in the context of low-glycaemic index dietary patterns on body weight and markers of adiposity: a systematic review and meta-analysis of randomised controlled trials in adults." *British Medical Journal Open* 2018 Apr 2;8(3):e019438.

32. Willcox BJ, Willcox DC. "Caloric restriction, caloric restriction mimetics, and healthy aging in Okinawa: controversies and clinical implications." *Current Opinion in Clinical Nutrition and Metabolic Care* 2014;17:51–58.

33. Mozaffarian D, Hao T, Rimm EB, Willett WC, Hu FB. "Changes in diet and lifestyle and long-term weight gain in women and men." *New England Journal of Medicine* 2011;364:2392–2404.

Chapter 3. Foods That Are Less Healthful Than You'd Think

1. Song M, Fung TT, Hu FB, et al. "Association of animal and plant protein intake with all-cause and cause-specific mortality." *JAMA Internal Medicine* 2016;176(10):1453–1463.

2. Naghshi S, Sadeghi O, Willett WC, Esmaillzadeh A. "Dietary intake of total, animal, and plant proteins and risk of all cause, cardiovascular, and cancer mortality: systematic review and dose-response meta-analysis of prospective cohort studies." *British Medical Journal* 2020;370:m2412.

3. Katz DL, Doughty KN, Geagan K, Jenkins DA, Gardner CD. "Perspective: the public health case for modernizing the definition of protein quality." *Advances in Nutrition* 2019;10:755–764.

4. Kakkoura MG, Du H, Guo Y, et al. "Dairy consumption and risks of total and site-specific cancers in Chinese adults: an 11-year prospective study of 0.5 million people." *BMC Medicine* 2022 May 6;20(1):134.

5. Fraser GE, Jaceldo-Siegl K, Orlich M, Mashchak A, Sirirat R, Knutsen S. "Dairy, soy, and risk of breast cancer: those confounded milks." *International Journal of Epidemiology* 2020;49:1526–1537.

6. Chan JM, Stampfer MJ, Ma J, Gann PH, Gaziano JM, Giovannucci EL. "Dairy products, calcium, and prostate cancer risk in the Physicians' Health Study." *American Journal of Clinical Nutrition* 2001;74(4):549–554.

7. David LA, Maurice CF, Carmody RN, et al. "Diet rapidly and reproducibly alters the human gut microbiome." *Nature* 2014;505(7484):559–563.

8. Barnard ND, Long MB, Ferguson JM, Flores R, Kahleova H. "Industry funding and cholesterol research: a systematic review." *American Journal of Lifestyle Medicine* 2019 Dec 11;15(2):165–172.

9. Rueda JM, Khosla P. "Impact of breakfasts (with or without eggs) on body weight regulation and blood lipids in university students over a 14-week semester." *Nutrients* 2013;5(12):5097–5113.

10. Barnard ND, Alwarith J, Rembert E, et al. "A Mediterranean diet and low-fat vegan diet to improve body weight and cardiometabolic risk factors: a randomized, cross-over trial." *Journal of the American College of Nutrition* 2021 Feb 5:1–13.

11. USDA Food Data Central. Avocados, California, raw. https://fdc.nal.usda.gov/fdc-app.html#/food-details/171706/nutrients, accessed April 7, 2023.

12. Lichtenstein AH, Kris-Etherton PM, Petersen KS, et al. "Effect of incorporating 1 avocado per day versus habitual diet on visceral adiposity: a randomized trial." *Journal of the American Heart Association* 2022 Jul 19;11(14):e025657.

13. Neelakantan N, Seah JYH, van Dam RM. "The effect of coconut oil consumption on cardiovascular risk factors: a systematic review and meta-analysis of clinical trials." *Circulation* 2020;141:803–814.

14. Sun Y, Neelakantan N, Wu Y, Lote-Oke R, Pan A, van Dam RM. "Palm oil consumption increases LDL cholesterol compared with vegetable oils low in saturated fat in a meta-analysis of clinical trials." *Journal of Nutrition* 2015;145:1549–1558.

15. Singh P, Arora A, Strand TA, et al. "Global prevalence of celiac disease: systematic review and meta-analysis." *Clinical Gastroenterology and Hepatology* 2018;16:823–836.

16. Tsilas CS, et al. "Relation of total sugars, fructose and sucrose with incident type 2 diabetes: a systematic review and meta-analysis of prospective cohort studies." *Canadian Medical Association Journal* 2017;189:E711–720.

17. Witkowski M, Nemet I, Alamri H, et al. "The artificial sweetener erythritol and cardiovascular event risk." *Nature Medicine* 2023. Feb 27. Epub ahead of print.

18. Lucerón-Lucas-Torres M, Cavero-Redondo I, Martínez-Vizcaíno V, Saz-Lara A, Pascual-Morena C, Álvarez-Bueno C. "Association between wine consumption and cognitive decline in older people: a systematic review and meta-analysis of longitudinal studies." *Frontiers in Nutrition* 2022;9:863059.

19. Zhao J, Stockwell T, Naimi T, Churchill S, Clay J, Sherk A. "Association between daily alcohol intake and risk of all-cause mortality: a systematic review and meta-analyses." *JAMA Network Open* 2023;6(3):e236185.

20. Krikorian R, Nash TA, Shidler MD, Shukitt-Hale B, Joseph JA. "Concord grape juice supplementation improves memory function in older adults with mild cognitive impairment." *British Journal of Nutrition* 2010;103:730–734.

21. Krikorian R, Skelton MR, Summer SS, Shidler MD, Sullivan PG. "Blueberry supplementation in midlife for dementia risk reduction." *Nutrients* 2022 Apr 13;14(8):1619.

Chapter 4. Drugs and Money

1. Palmer SC, Tendal B, Mustafa RA, et al. "Sodium-glucose cotransporter protein-2 (SGLT-2) inhibitors and glucagon-like peptide-1 (GLP-1) receptor agonists for type 2 diabetes: systematic review and network meta-analysis of randomised controlled trials." *British Medical Journal* 2021 Jan 13;372:m4573; Huynh G, Runeberg H, Weideman R. "Evaluating weight loss with semaglutide in elderly patients with type II diabetes." *Journal of Pharmacy Technology* 2023 Feb;39(1):10–15.

2. Wilding JPH, Batterham RL, Calanna S, et al. "Once-weekly semaglutide in adults with overweight or obesity." *New England Journal of Medicine* 2021;384(11):989–1002; Tan HC, Dampil OA, Marquez MM. "Efficacy and safety of semaglutide for weight loss in obesity without diabetes: a systematic review and meta-analysis." *Journal of the ASEAN Federation of Endocrine Societies* 2022;37:65–72.

3. Bezin J, Gouverneur A, Pénichon M, et al. "GLP-1 receptor agonists and the risk of thyroid cancer." *Diabetes Care* 2023;46(2):384–390.

4. Wilding JPH, Batterham RL, Davies M, et al. "Weight regain and cardiometabolic effects after withdrawal of semaglutide: the STEP 1 trial extension." *Diabetes, Obesity and Metabolism* 2022;24:1553–1564.

5. Weiss T, Carr RD, Pal S, et al. "Real-world adherence and discontinuation of glucagon-like peptide-1 receptor agonists therapy in type 2 diabetes mellitus patients in the United States." *Patient Preference and Adherence* 2020 Nov 27;14:2337–2345.

6. Weiss T, Yang L, Carr RD, et al. "Real-world weight change, adherence, and discontinuation among patients with type 2 diabetes initiating glucagon-like peptide-1 receptor agonists in the UK." *BMJ Open Diabetes Research Care* 2022 Jan;10(1):e002517.

7. Leach J, Chodroff M, Qiu Y, Leslie RS, Urick B, Marshall L, Gleason P.

"Real-world analysis of glucagon-like peptide-1 agonist (GLP-1a) obesity treatment one year cost-effectiveness and therapy adherence." Prime Therapeutics, July 11, 2023. Available at: https://www.primetherapeutics.com/wp-content /uploads/2023/07/GLP-1a-obesity-treatment-1st-year-cost-effectiveness-study -abstract-FINAL-7-11.pdf.

8. Weiss T, Yang L, Carr RD, et al. "Real-world weight change, adherence, and discontinuation among patients with type 2 diabetes initiating glucagon-like peptide-1 receptor agonists in the UK." *BMJ Open Diabetes Research and Care* 2022 Jan;10(1):e002517.

9. Prime Therapeutics. "Real-world analysis of GLP-1a drugs for weight loss finds low adherence and increased cost in first year." July 11, 2023. Available at: https://www.primetherapeutics.com/news/real-world-analysis-of-glp-1a-drugs -for-weight-loss-finds-low-adherence-and-increased-cost-in-first-year/.

10. Bodnaruc AM, Prud'homme D, Blanchet R, Giroux I. "Nutritional modulation of endogenous glucagon-like peptide-1 secretion: a review." *Nutrition and Metabolism (London)* 2016;13:92.

11. Belinova L, Kahleova H, Malinska H, et al. "Differential acute postprandial effects of processed meat and isocaloric vegan meals on the gastrointestinal hormone response in subjects suffering from type 2 diabetes and healthy controls: a randomized crossover study." *PLoS ONE* 2014;9(9):e107561; Herman GA, Bergman A, Stevens C, et al. "Effect of single oral doses of sitagliptin, a dipeptidyl peptidase-4 inhibitor, on incretin and plasma glucose levels after an oral glucose tolerance test in patients with type 2 diabetes." *Journal of Clinical Endocrinology and Metabolism* 2006;91:4612–4619.

12. Kahleova H, Tura A, Klementova M, et al. "A plant-based meal stimulates incretin and insulin secretion more than an energy- and macronutrient-matched standard meal in type 2 diabetes: a randomized crossover study." *Nutrients* 2019;11:486.

13. Diagram adapted from Belinova L, Kahleova H, Malinska H, et al. "Differential acute postprandial effects of processed meat and isocaloric vegan meals on the gastrointestinal hormone response in subjects suffering from type 2 diabetes and healthy controls: a randomized crossover study." *PLoS ONE* 2014;9(9):e107561. Used by permission.

14. Khandelwal S, Zemore SE, Hemmerling A. "Nutrition education in internal medicine residency programs and predictors of residents' dietary counseling practices." *Journal of Medical Education and Curricular Development* 2018 5;2382120518763360.

15. Singh P, Zhang Y, Sharma P, Covassin N, Soucek F, Friedman PA, Somers VK. "Statins decrease leptin expression in human white adipocytes." *Physiological Reports* 2018 Jan;6(2):e13566.

16. Swerdlow DI, Preiss D, Kuchenbaecker KB, et al. "HMG-coenzyme A reductase inhibition, type 2 diabetes, and bodyweight: evidence from genetic analysis and randomised trials." *Lancet* 2015;385(9965):351–361.

17. Alvarez-Jimenez L, Morales-Palomo F, Moreno-Cabañas A, Ortega JF, Mora-Rodríguez R. "Effects of statin therapy on glycemic control and insulin

resistance: a systematic review and meta-analysis." *European Journal of Pharmacology* 2023 Mar 24;947:175672; Sattar N, Preiss D, Murray HM, et al. "Statins and risk of incident diabetes: a collaborative meta-analysis of randomised statin trials." *Lancet* 2010;375(9716):735–742.

18. Sugiyama T, Tsugawa Y, Tseng CH, Kobayashi Y, Shapiro MF. "Different time trends of caloric and fat intake between statin users and nonusers among US adults: gluttony in the time of statins?" *JAMA Internal Medicine* 2014;174:1038–1045.

19. UK Prospective Diabetes Study (UKPDS) Group. "Intensive blood-glucose control with sulphonylureas or insulin compared with conventional treatment and risk of complications in patients with type 2 diabetes (UKPDS 33)." *Lancet* 1998;352(9131):837–853.

Chapter 5. Meal Planning for Breakfast, Lunch, Dinner, and Snacks

1. Meyer HE, Willett WC, Fung TT, Holvik K, Feskanich D. "Association of high intakes of vitamins B6 and B12 from food and supplements with risk of hip fracture among postmenopausal women in the Nurses' Health Study." *JAMA Network Open* 2019 May 3;2(5):e193591.

2. Song M, Fung TT, Hu FB, et al. "Association of animal and plant protein intake with all-cause and cause-specific mortality." *JAMA Internal Medicine* 2016;176:1453–1463.

3. Naghshi S, Sadeghi O, Willett WC, Esmaillzadeh A. "Dietary intake of total, animal, and plant proteins and risk of all cause, cardiovascular, and cancer mortality: systematic review and dose-response meta-analysis of prospective cohort studies." *British Medical Journal* 2020;370:m2412.

Chapter 6. Eating on the Go

1. The Agricultural Marketing Act of 1946. 7 U.S.C. § 1622(e)(1).

Chapter 7. Go for the Max

1. Solomon A, Kivipelto M, Wolozin B, Zhou J, Whitmer RA. "Midlife serum cholesterol and increased risk of Alzheimer's and vascular dementia three decades later." *Dementia and Geriatric Cognitive Disorders* 2009;28:75–80.

2. Barnard ND, Cohen J, Jenkins DJ, Turner-McGrievy G, Gloede L, Jaster B, Seidl K, Green AA, Talpers S. "A low-fat vegan diet improves glycemic control and cardiovascular risk factors in a randomized clinical trial in individuals with type 2 diabetes." *Diabetes Care* 2006 Aug;29(8):1777–1783.

3. Beezhold BL, Johnston CS. "Restriction of meat, fish, and poultry in omnivores improves mood: a pilot randomized controlled trial." *Nutrition Journal* 2012;11:9; Ferdowsian HR, Barnard ND, Hoover VJ, Katcher HI, Levin SM, Green AA, Cohen JL. "A multi-component intervention reduces body weight and cardiovascular risk at a GEICO corporate site." *American Journal of Health Promotion* 2010;24:384–387; Katcher HI, Ferdowsian HR, Hoover

VJ, Cohen JL, Barnard ND. "A worksite vegan nutrition program is well-accepted and improves health-related quality of life and work productivity." *Annals of Nutrition and Metabolism* 2010;56:245–252; Mishra S, Xu J, Agarwal U, Gonzales J, Levin S, Barnard N. "A multicenter randomized controlled trial of a plant-based nutrition program to reduce body weight and cardiovascular risk in the corporate setting: the GEICO study." *European Journal of Clinical Nutrition* 2013;67:718–724; Agarwal U, Mishra S, Xu J, Levin S, Gonzales J, Barnard N. "A multicenter randomized controlled trial of a nutrition intervention program in a multiethnic adult population in the corporate setting reduces depression and anxiety and improves quality of life: the GEICO Study." *American Journal of Health Promotion* 2015;29(4):245–254.

4. Barnard ND, Noble EP, Ritchie T, et al. "D2 dopamine receptor Taq1A polymorphism, body weight, and dietary intake in type 2 diabetes." *Nutrition* 2009;25:58–65.

Index

About the Author

Neal Barnard, MD, FACC, is an adjunct professor of medicine at the George Washington University School of Medicine in Washington, DC, and founder and president of the Physicians Committee for Responsible Medicine.

Dr. Barnard has led numerous research studies investigating the effects of diet on diabetes, body weight, hormonal symptoms, and chronic pain, including a groundbreaking study of dietary interventions in type 2 diabetes, funded by the National Institutes of Health, that paved the way for viewing type 2 diabetes as a potentially reversible condition for many patients. Dr. Barnard has authored more than one hundred scientific publications and twenty books for medical and lay readers and is the editor-in-chief of the *Nutrition Guide for Clinicians*, a textbook made available to all US medical students.

As president of the Physicians Committee, Dr. Barnard leads programs advocating for preventive medicine, good nutrition, and higher ethical standards in research. In 2015, he was named a Fellow of the American College of Cardiology. In 2016, he founded the Barnard Medical Center in Washington, DC, as a model for making nutrition a routine part of all medical care.

Working with the Medical Society of the District of Columbia and the American Medical Association, Dr. Barnard has authored key resolutions, now part of AMA policy, calling for a new focus on prevention and nutrition in federal policies and in medical practice. In 2018, he received the Medical Society of the District of Columbia's

Distinguished Service Award. He has hosted four PBS television programs on nutrition and health.

Originally from Fargo, North Dakota, Dr. Barnard received his MD degree at the George Washington University School of Medicine and completed his residency at the same institution. He practiced at St. Vincent's Hospital in New York before returning to Washington to found the Physicians Committee.